Multiple Choice Questions for the MRCPsych

Part II Basic Sciences Examination

To Simrit, Suvinder and Saj (aka Bob)

Multiple Choice Questions for the MRCPsych

Part II Basic Sciences Examination

Gin S. Malhi MB ChB BSc(Hons) MRCPsych
Clinical Lecturer, Institute of Psychiatry, Maudsley Hospital, London, UK

Foreword by
Professor David Goldberg
Professor of Psychiatry, Institute of Psychiatry, London

A member of the Hodder Headline Group
LONDON • NEW YORK • NEW DELHI

This edition first published in Great Britain in 2000 by Butterworth Heinemann.

This impression published in 2002 by
Arnold, a member of the Hodder Headline Group,
338 Euston Road, London NW1 3BH

http://www.arnoldpublishers.com

Distributed in the USA by
Oxford University Press Inc.,
198 Madison Avenue, New York, NY10016
Oxford is a registered trademark of Oxford University Press

Whilst the advice and information in this book are believed to be true and
accurate at the date of going to press, neither the authors nor the publisher
can accept any legal responsibility or liability for any errors or omissions
that may be made. In particular (but without limiting the generality of the
preceding disclaimer) every effort has been made to check drug dosages;
however, it is still possible that errors have been missed. Furthermore,
dosage schedules are constantly being revised and new side-effects
recognized. For these reasons the reader is strongly urged to consult the
drug companies' printed instructions before administering any of the drugs
recommended in this book.

British Library Cataloguing in Publication Data
A catalogue record for this book is available from the British Library

Library of Congress Cataloging-in-Publication Data
A catalog record for this book is available from the Library of Congress

ISBN 0 7506 4089 8

1 2 3 4 5 6 7 8 9 10

Printed and bound in India by Replika Press PVT Ltd

What do you think about this book? Or any other Arnold title?
Please send your comments to feedback.arnold@hodder.co.uk

Contents

Foreword to series

As the authors rightly say in Chapter 4, for most candidates examinations are an ordeal – disruptive, onerous, worrying and tedious. Nothing can be done to remove the anxiety completely, to banish the burden, or to eliminate the tedium. However, in so far as anything can lighten the candidate's burden or to replace terror with hope, these books are it.

When the College was first set up, the old Royal Medico-Psychological Association sought to model itself on the College of Physicians of London, which at that time made rather little effort to maintain standards of training posts, but expended much effort on devising a punitive examination with a very high failure rate. A deputation of dissidents from the Maudsley protested about these plans, and demanded that the new College should have a major concern with ensuring that candidates for the future examination received a proper clinical training. Two members of this deputation were later to become President of the College and Chief Examiner, and I think that all the others have served the College as Examiners.

The College has a proud record in having ensured that training schemes were set up in such a way that young psychiatrists receive a balanced training, and that consultants take their teaching responsibilities seriously. Unlike most other colleges, ours has a nationwide system of clinical tutors charged with specific responsibilities towards trainees. This being so, one cannot complain if the College also sets a searching professional examination for its potential members.

In the years since the College was set up there have been enormous advances in our understanding of both basic and clinical neuroscience, and less dramatic but still substantial advances in knowledge in social psychiatry. The most demanding test of this knowledge is embodied in the three multiple choice question (MCQ) examinations set by the College.

Foreword

These books do three things well: they acquaint the candidate with examples of up-to-date test material across the entire range of the examination; they increase the candidate's knowledge by giving informative answers accompanied by references to original papers dealing with the test materials, and they shamelessly teach candidates the tricks of the trade to ensure that they get the highest possible mark for the level of knowledge that they in fact possess by the time the examination comes round.

In reading through the test material that makes up the bulk of these three volumes I have been impressed by how much I learned myself. I had thought that I had kept up with my reading since the time when I completed my own examinations — but often when I strayed from my own areas of special interest I found that I was learning new material by attempting the test material and then checking my responses against the helpful notes that follow on the next page.

Those who work their way through this book are likely to emerge as better-informed psychiatrists. If they have to sit the MCQ examination, they will undoubtedly obtain a much higher score than before. It seems almost unfair — but there is nothing improper about it.

Professor David Goldberg
Professor of Psychiatry, Institute of Psychiatry

Preface

The *Multiple Choice Questions in Psychiatry* series comprises three volumes – one for each of the three MCQ papers in the MRCPsych examination. This volume is designed to prepare candidates for the MRCPsych Part II Basic Sciences paper; the other two volumes are for the MRCPsych Part I multiple choice examination paper and the MRCPsych Part II clinical topics paper. Section I of each book is similar and is tailored to the particular examination being addressed.

The MCQ papers, like other components of the MRCPsych examination, require practice and adequate preparation. Candidates sitting Part II of the MRCPsych examination will have passed Part I and should have sufficient clinical knowledge and experience to at least tackle most components of the examination. However, the basic science paper covers topics that most candidates will need to revise and perhaps learn. Multiple choice questions by their very nature allow testing of very specific knowledge and it is important therefore not to underestimate the amount of preparation necessary. This book has been written in conjunction with the *Examination Notes in Psychiatry Basic Sciences* text. However, neither of these are a substitute for reading widely.

The multiple choice questions in this book are drawn from discussions with candidates who have recently sat the MRCPsych Part II papers. They have been scrutinized by candidates preparing for the examination, those that have passed and also those that have failed. All the multiple choice questions have been assessed in terms of composition, relevance and difficulty. However, there may still be errors and so candidates are advised to check answers particularly if an answer invokes doubts.

I am grateful to the many candidates who have helped develop the questions in this book but I am particularly indebted to my own 'psychiatry teachers' (Dr German Berrios, Dr Paul Bridges, Professor David Goldberg, Dr Frank Holloway, Dr Rob Howard and Dr Veronica O'Keane), who imbued me with a passion for learning.

Gin S. Malhi

Section I

1

How to use this book

This book, like its sister volumes in the *Multiple Choice Questions in Psychiatry* series, has been prepared with the following aims in mind:

1. To provide instruction on the principles and intentions behind the setting of MCQs in the hope that you will derive information that will be of assistance in answering this form of question.
2. To provide advice and guidance on the nature of the MRCPsych Part II examination and on aspects of the regulations.
3. To equip you with the expertise and skills with which to answer MCQs.
4. To supply you with advice on how to organize and carry out your revision.
5. To provide practice examination papers that will enable you to rehearse your technique, assess your knowledge and acquire new knowledge.

This first section contains important preparatory chapters and it is strongly recommended that these are studied carefully before the examination papers are attempted. Chapter 2 contains an outline of the nature of the MRCPsych Part II examination, and the third chapter is designed to better your understanding of MCQs – the principles used in their construction and the implications of certain terms that they commonly contain. The fourth chapter considers how to revise for the examination, and discusses how to take the examination. Section I concludes with an important résumé of the rules and principles that you should use both to prepare for the examination and to sit it.

In Section II the practice MCQ questions are arranged into five mock examination papers.

The answers contain useful explanatory notes that will enhance your knowledge.

The composition of the practice examination papers reflects the syllabus published in the regulations published by the Royal College of Psychiatrists.

2

The MRCPsych Part II examination

Information

General information and regulations for the MRCPsych examinations are published by the Royal College of Psychiatrists. Since these are subject to regular amendment, *the candidate is strongly advised to write to the College for the most current regulations.* Ensure you know the closing dates for complete applications well in advance; many candidates apply in a last-minute rush; inevitably some miss the date. Application forms are available on written request to the Examinations Department.

The address of the Royal College of Psychiatrists is:

The Royal College of Psychiatrists
17 Belgrave Square
London
SW1X 8PG

The entry requirements for the MRCPsych Part II

The Royal College of Psychiatrists publishes details of the registration requirements for entry to the examination and these should be referred to in general, suitably registered candidates must have passed the MRCPsych Part I or have obtained exemption from it. Candidates are normally expected to have fulfilled 3 years of full-time (or equivalent part-time) training in a post-registration training scheme that has College approval. The College publishes helpful guidelines on what constitutes approved training, and what 'credit' can be gained from, for example, completing postgraduate degrees, foreign training and postgraduate medical training. Ensure you obtain the current regulations and know the entry requirements at the beginning of your training, not when you are about to apply to sit the examination. Candidates must also comply with the regulations concerning registration and sponsorship. Finally, should you have to withdraw before an examination, note very carefully the College's regulations regarding the procedure it accepts.

Sponsorship

On each occasion that the examination is attempted candidates are expected to furnish sponsorship forms confirming that they have had satisfactory training available in a range of specified areas. Statements are required from two sponsors therefore make sure you identify them in good time.

Components of the MRCPsych Part II examination

The Part II examination consists of the following elements (Royal College of Psychiatrists, 1994):

1. Two MCQ papers: (N.B. Negative marking is no longer used)
   Sciences basic to psychiatry (1 ½ hours, 50 questions)
   Clinical topics (1 ½ hours, 50 questions)
2. One essay paper
   (1 ½ hours, two assays to be written)
3. One Critical Review Paper
4. On clinical examination
   (1 ½ hours: a 1-hour 'long case' and a half-hour afterwards with a pair of examiners)
5. One patient management problem oral examination
   (½ hour)

Number of attempts allowed at the MRCPsych Part II

Five attempts are allowed at this examination. Candidates who fail on their second, third or fourth attempt are not allowed to resit until they have had a further 6 months of full-time (or equivalent part-time) approved training.

The pass mark

The Royal College has said that to pass the MRCPsych Part II a candidate 'must pass the Clinical Examination and achieve a standard in the other sections which is acceptable to the Examinations Sub-Committee' (Royal College of Psychiatrists, 1993).

Officers of the College have stated: 'the marking of the MRCPsych examinations and the establishment of pass criteria are complex and confidential. We want to make it clear however that there is no single pass mark derived from the MCQ papers, and candidates should not base their examination technique on such an assumption. They should, quite simply, aim to score as high as possible.

Summary

1. Current examination regulations are available through a written application to the Examination Department of the Royal College of Psychiatrists.
2. The entry requirements should be studied early in your training, not just before you apply.
3. Identify your potential sponsors and understand their role.
4. Ensure you understand how you are going to be examined. Orient your learning to this.

3

The multiple choice question

It is of considerable advantage when preparing for an MCQ examination to understand how MCQs are constructed. Of the many sources available for this purpose, the account by Anderson (1976) remains the most authoritative and useful. Much of the following information on the MCQ is based on this account.

Why use MCQs at all?

The MCQ format grew out of a need to have an objective method to assess and rank candidates and has been the subject of debate by John Anderson and Sir George Pickering (Anderson, 1979, 1981; Pickering, 1979).

Unlike essays and orals, the well-constructed MCQ examination paper excludes the subjective bias of examiners and ensures all candidates are examined on the same material. Candidates are discouraged from hasty guessing by the adoption of negative marking – the deduction of a mark for an incorrect response. This is a stratagem that also simplifies the process of discriminating between candidates.

It should be emphasized that the well-constructed MCQ paper is an ideal to which examination authors aspire but often fail to achieve, since there are many pitfalls; the experience of sitting on examination committees that review questions quickly shows that it is not at all uncommon for questions to advance into examination papers still imperfect in one respect or another. Furthermore, not all knowledge areas in psychiatry lend themselves to examination by MCQ (Strauss *et al.*, 1982).

What principles do examiners follow when constructing MCQs and can knowledge of these principles be of assistance to you?

The brief answer to this is that examiners seek to produce well-constructed questions in plain English that follow the syllabus and discriminate adequately between candidates of varying ability. There are certain rules or principles and in some circumstances, as we shall see, if you are knowledgeable about the setting of MCQs you can use stylistic errors and grammatical clues to your advantage.

What are the various components of MCQ questions called?

There is a set of precise terms that are used to describe the component parts of the MCQ and it is well worth getting to know them. These are given in Table 1.

Table 1 Definitions of terms used to describe aspects of the MCQ

Term	Definition
True	One of the three recognized responses to a question. Such a response may be correct or incorrect; true and correct are not synonymous
False	One of the three recognized responses to a question. Such a response may be correct or incorrect; false and incorrect are not synonymous
Don't know	One of the three recognized responses to a question. No marks are awarded or deducted for using this response
Stem	The introductory statement which, together with an option, forms one of the five component questions of an MCQ
Option	The stem is followed by five options, labelled A to E. Each option (sometimes called a *completion*) will, in combination with the stem, form a discrete question, known as an item. Each of the five items in a given MCQ is independent of the other four
Item	The stem and option together form an item. In College examinations a given MCQ will contain five component items
Distractor	An item for which the correct response is *False*

Modified from Anderson (1976)

9

Use of English

MCQs should employ plain English that is precise and to the point. Unfortunately, where this is not achieved, you may face ambiguity or, where English is not your first language, actual disadvantage.

Breadth and depth of the questions

The examination should be set to reflect the syllabus and the questions pitched at an appropriate level of difficulty. From the examiners' point of view, if the questions are too easy, the scores will not discriminate between candidates of varying calibre. If you have an especially advanced knowledge of a particular topic, you should not overread the question; that is, you should assume the examiners are setting it at the level of a good to advanced clinician, not that of an advanced research worker. Many candidates create ambiguity in their minds in this way, and if you find this happening, you need to muse on what the examiners' intention was.

At the level of specialist medical examinations, examiners are rarely devious and should be trusted.

Certain words and phrases crop up regularly in MCQs – should they be interpreted in a particular way?

Some words and phrases (Table 2) do have a generally accepted usage and therefore you must be familiar with them. Question practice will help considerably. Vigilance is required and if there is plenty of time left at the end, double-check your interpretation of any question item containing these words and phrases.

Negatives require a special mention. Examiners usually avoid them, but inevitably they creep in, often when there is a need to make the correct response to an item a little less obvious. Approach negatives, especially double-negatives, with caution and, again, you might check you have interpreted them correctly if there is time at the end of the examination.

The word 'may' still appears in the wording of MCQs, despite criticism of its use (Bisson, 1991). Essentially the word 'may' implies a possibility, however remote, and thus True is likely to be the correct answer, though not always. Absolute words such as 'always' and 'never' are usually avoided by examiners, as the correct response is so rarely anything but False. if you come across these you will usually be correct to guess False; those few where True really is the correct answer will hopefully be apparent to you.

Table 2 Definitions of words widely used in the stems and options of MCQ questions

Word	Definition
Characteristic	A word that has a specific meaning – a characteristic feature is a feature that would be expected to occur for the diagnosis to be made, and where absent would lead to some doubt about the diagnosis
Commonly	A term that should be taken to mean an event that occurs more than 50% of the time
Pathognomonic	A pathognomonic feature implies the feature being referred to occurs in the disease or disorder named only, and in no other
Recognized	A recognized feature is a feature of a disorder that has been reported and which a candidate would reasonably be expected to know of. Characteristic features are always recognized, but the reverse may not be the case
Specific	A term generally used in the same way as pathognomonic
Typical	A term that should be taken as a synonym for characteristic

Modified from Anderson (1976)

Slade and Dewey (1983) have studied the role of grammatical clues in MCQ examinations and reach interesting conclusions.

By scrutinizing the sample paper of the old Preliminary Test of the Royal College of Psychiatrists, a list of 34 words and phrases was produced which it was felt contained grammatical features that tended to discriminate between True and False response items (Table 3).

The authors looked to see if these grammatical clues could be applied to MCQs other than those from which they were derived. They could, and with some considerable benefit. It was found that 18% of a random sample of 600 question items in a widely used MCQ book could be responded to from grammatical clues alone, and almost four-fifths of these (80 out of 107) would have been answered correctly. They went on to show that subjects do obtain higher scores on items that contain grammatical clues, particularly where they are contained in the option.

As in practice it is hard to set MCQ papers free from grammatical clues, it would seem that the candidate who is aware of these clues, and uses this knowledge *with care*, could potentially raise the score he or she has derived from factual knowledge alone – potentially taking the score over the threshold of a pass.

Table 3 Positive and negative key words and phrases

True responses	False responses
May	Always
May be	Necessarily
Can be	Is necessarily
Can appear	Characteristically
Tend(s)	Typically
Contribute to	All
Is of benefit	First
Of value	Appropriate
Useful	Same as
Suggest(s)	The fact that
Is possible	Do(es) not
Encourages	Requires
Are (is) often	No value
Are (is) frequently	Are free from
Have (has) been	Is complete
Usually	Very useful
	Is important
	Essential

From Slade and Dewey (1993), with permission.
Note: this table is included to illustrate the research discussed in the test. It should not be assumed that these words can be used in the examination to predict what the correct response might be.

Precision with terms

Examiners seek to set clear questions, but imprecision can slip in unnoticed. For example, the term schizophrenia may be used without qualification as to what subtype, if any, is being referred to. Rather than leave the question out, once again you should trust that the examiner is not being devious.

Eponymous names, while not necessarily unfair are best qualified in brackets; where not, the examiner may often be relied upon to have left a clue to the disorder in the options supplied. Drug doses or percentages may be stated in a way that implies that a figure differing by a small amount would be wrong. You may realize such precision is wrong and be tempted to use the response Don't Know because of the ambiguity created. It is better, however, just to accept the examiner's slip and assume the figure to be correct if it is in the right area. You should feel justifiably aggrieved if only the trade name of a drug is given – in practice, however, this is most unlikely to occur.

Summary

1. There is a generally accepted set of principles governing the setting of MCQ questions. It is advantageous to understand these rule.
2. Take the time to learn the definition of terms such as item, distractor and stem.
3. Avoid overreading the difficulty of questions – become familiar with the general standard required by your examiners.
4. Learn the meaning of terms such as characteristic, typical and recognized.
5. Familiarize yourself with the correct interpretation of words and phrases that may provide grammatical clues.
6. Care is required not only in interpreting terms that have been used with excessive precision but also with those that are used imprecisely.

4

Passing the examination

How to prepare for the examination

By the time you come to sit the MRCPsych Part II, you should be relatively experienced at examination preparation and the following sections may at first seem superfluous. However, if revising, surely it is just as logical to revise your technique as well as the facts themselves? Thus, read the following sections carefully at the outset, and refer to them again once you are underway.

When to start your revision?

Individuals will vary in the time they give to their revision. Six months seems about right for most – any longer and you may find it hard to sustain your interest, any less and the task may be more of a struggle. It is beneficial to try to be ready 2 weeks before the exam – in practice this will be liable to slip to a week or less.

What books to use?

Use a few core texts but know them well. The books listed in 'suggested reading' are suitable texts for the basic sciences aspect of the MRCPsych Part II. Avoid the tendency to consult too many sources, with the risk of ending up with a bewildering collection of barely used books. There can be little doubt that if those listed are systematically studied then you will be left with few gaps.

How to get organized?

Careful attention to the organization of your revision will be of huge value to you. For each aspect of the Part II examination you should devise a revision strategy. It will become immediately apparent that there is a lot to do. It is important to set targets or time will fritter away in inefficient study. Balance is required – for example, it will be of little help to know phenomenology inside out, if the rest of the syllabus is neglected. You may have to compromise on your initial objectives – corners will have to be cut and material left out.

What to do for the MCQ Basic Sciences paper?

As mentioned above, the preparation for this MCQ paper should be integrated into your total revision programme. Much of the factual knowledge will accumulate from the reading that you have undertaken. After first devoting time to studying MCQ question technique, you should get lots of practice in doing questions. Your adeptness at doing MCQs will increase, as will your factual base, especially if you use MCQs that are supplied with explanatory answers and references. You should ideally make brief notes of new pieces of information. Arrange these under the main headings in the syllabus, allowing a sheet of paper for each heading. It is especially advantageous for you to sit practice examinations such as those contained in this book. As you do this, assess your technique as well as your factual knowledge. Technique is considered in detail below.

How to approach the last 2 weeks?

As mentioned earlier, it is ideal to have completed your revision about 2 weeks before the examinations. In the last 2 weeks review areas of difficulty, look through any notes you have highlighted for final revision and rehearse your examination technique.

Summary

1. It is ideal to approach your revision with a foundation of steady learning behind you. Start your revision in good time and aim to leave some time over before the examinations for more leisurely final revision.
2. Stick to a small number of core texts but know them thoroughly.
3. Integrate your revision for the various sections of the Part II examination within a well-organized timetable. Set yourself deadlines and keep to them.
4. Do large numbers of MCQs, especially as complete papers under examination conditions. Make brief notes of new pieces of

information.
5. Give time and thought to your psychological preparation. Above all, avoid getting overtired and inefficient.
6. It is advantageous, but not essential, to attend a revision course. Leave time for this in your timetable, completing most of your revision before you arrive on the course.
7. Use your last 2 weeks to consolidate your learning.

In the examination – how best to approach doing the MCQ paper?

General points

Read over the instructions, however familiar they may appear. Ensure you understand how many questions there are to do in what period (in the MRCPsych Part II this should of course be 50 questions in 90 minutes).

As you go through the paper, ensure you have placed your answers on the response sheet in the correct place; if you miss a question out there is a risk of muddling up the subsequent numbering. Check that all your responses are clearly marked in the spaces provided.

Which method to employ in answering the questions?

As there is no fixed pass mark your objective is to score as many marks as possible. Thus, don't stop when you believe you have correctly answered enough to score at a hypothetical pass mark.

Summary

1. Read the examination instructions carefully.
2. Always check that you have placed your answers on the response sheet correctly and ensure that the lozenges are clearly marked.
3. Read the items carefully. Use the technique for answering the questions which previous rehearsal has shown suits you best.

References

Anderson, J. (1976) *The Multiple Choice Question in Medicine*. Tunbridge Wells: Pitman Medical.

Anderson, J. (1979) For multiple choice questions. *Medical Teacher* 1, 37.

Anderson, J. (1981) The MCQ controversy – a review. *Medical Teacher* 3, 150–156.

Bisson, J.I. (1991) The psychiatric MCQ: are "possibles" always true? *Psychiatric Bulletin* 15, 90–91.

Pickering, G. (1979) Against multiple choice questions. *Medical Teacher* 1, 84.

Royal College of Psychiatrists (1994) *General Information and Regulations for the MRCPsych Examinations*. London: Royal College of Psychiatrists.

Slade, P.D. & Dewey, M.E. (1983) Role of grammatical clues in multiple choice questions: an empirical study. *Medical Teacher* 5, 146–148. Published by Taylor & Francis Ltd, http://www.tandf.co.uk

Strauss, G.D., Yager, J. & Strauss, G.E. (1982) Assessing assessment: the content and quality of the psychiatry in-training examination. *American Journal of Psychiatry* 139, 85–88.

Section II

Sample examination response sheets

Paper 1

1.1 Classical conditioning:
- A. Involves associative learning.
- B. Requires understanding.
- C. Is most effective if the conditioned and unconditioned stimuli are applied simultaneously.
- D. Is termed trace conditioning if the conditioned stimulus ends prior to the application of the unconditioned stimulus.
- E. Is unaffected by stimulus preparedness.

1.2 The following are true:
- A. Insight learning is a form of observational learning.
- B. Modelling is a form of observational learning.
- C. Latent learning is a form of cognitive learning.
- D. Vicarious learning is a form of associative learning.
- E. Respondent learning is a form of cognitive learning.

1.3 Visual development; at birth:
- A. Infant is able to track and scan objects.
- B. Depth perception is present.
- C. Infant can discriminate levels of brightness.
- D. Infant possesses perceptual constancy.
- E. Infant can differentiate figures against a uniform background (figure ground differentiation)

1.4 Memory:
- A. Sensory memory is of small capacity.
- B. Visual short-term memory is usually stored in the left hemisphere.
- C. Sensory memory usually lasts 20–30 s.
- D. Short-term memory fades unless rehearsed.
- E. Multi-store model of memory was described by Jouvet.

1.1

A. True – Both classical and operant conditioning are forms of associative learning.
B. False – The association is an automatic behaviour.
C. False – Simultaneous conditioning is less effective than delayed conditioning in which the conditioned stimulus precedes the unconditional stimulus. Note that the optimal delay is 0.5 s.
D. True – Least effective.
E. False – Stimulus preparedness: some stimuli are more likely to become a conditioned stimulus than others.

1.2

A. False – It is a type of cognitive learning.
B. True – Also called imitation learning. Takes place through observation.
C. True – Learning occurs but is not immediately apparent.
D. False – Another term for observational learning.
E. False – It is a type of associative learning better known as classical conditioning.

1.3

A. True.
B. False – Present at age 2 months.
C. True.
D. False – Perceptual constancy, depth perception and object completion are acquired abilities.
E. True.

1.4

A. False – Large capacity but of very brief duration.
B. False – It is usually stored in the right hemisphere.
C. False – This applies to short-term memory. Sensory memory lasts less than half a second.
D. True.
E. False – by Atkinson and Shiffrin.

1.5 Attitudes have specific functions; these include:
A. The expression of values.
B. Facilitating understanding of the world.
C. Preservation of self-esteem.
D. Engendering sense of belonging.
E. Promoting compromise.

1.6 The following measures are correctly described:
A. Likert scale – consists of paired bipolar adjectives.
B. Thurstone scale – consists of statements that have been ranked and assigned values.
C. Semantic differential scale – has good test–retest reliability.
D. Sociometry – involves subjects in groups nominating their preferred partners. This creates sociograms which are then used to identify sub-groups.
E. Raven's progressive matrices – rely on recall of information.

1.7 In Festinger's cognitive dissonance theory:
A. Dissonance arises because of inconsistency between attitudes and behaviour.
B. Dissonance is characterized by decreased arousal.
C. Dissonance is reduced by altering behaviour.
D. Dissonance is reduced by changing attitude.
E. Dissonance is reduced by dismissing information responsible for creating dissonance.

1.8 The Halstead–Reitan Neuropsychological Battery (HRNB):
A. Is used for diagnosing brain damage.
B. Includes the Wechsler Adult Intelligence Scale.
C. Can be completed in a matter of minutes.
D. Lacks normative data for psychiatric populations.
E. Has high discriminative accuracy.

1.5

    A. True – Value-expressive.
    B. True – Knowledge.
    C. True – Ego-defensive.
    D. True – Social adjustment.
    E. False.

Note: Attitudes are also instrumental.

1.6

    A. False – This describes a semantic differential scale. Likert scale comprises a number of statements and for each the subject indicates their degree of agreement/disagreement.
    B. True.
    C. True.
    D. True.
    E. False – They do not rely on information recall.

1.7

    A. True – This then usually leads to a change of attitudes so that they are consistent with behaviour.
    B. False – It is associated with increased arousal.
    C. True.
    D. True.
    E. True.

Note: Dissonance can also be countered by developing and adding new explanations or ideas in favour of thoughts that are consonant.

1.8

    A. True – It is one of the most commonly used batteries used for this purpose.
    B. True – It consists of 11 components including the WAIS, MMPI and Trail Making and Category Tests.
    C. False – It takes several hours to complete.
    D. False – There is normative data for psychiatric, organic and normal populations.
    E. True – It has a discriminative accuracy of more than 80%.

1.9 The following errors of assessment are correctly described:
A. Hawthorne effect: answers are selected so as to fit with other responses.
B. Response set: tendency to always agree or disagree with questions.
C. Leniency error: bias towards centre, avoiding extremes.
D. Halo effect: respondent gives answers believed to be expected by interviewer.
E. Logical error: tendency to select extremes.

1.10 Intelligence:
A. Is calculated as a quotient (IQ) by dividing chronological age by mental age.
B. Is divided by Sternberg into component and experiential intelligence.
C. Is denoted by '*g*' as a general factor of intelligence.
D. Steadily increases up to 35 years of age.
E. Exhibits a terminal drop 5 years prior to death.

1.11 In avoidant attachment behaviour:
A. In the absence of the attachment figure the child is excessively anxious.
B. Upon return of the attachment figure the child displays little or no reaction.
C. There is a likelihood of developing future aggressive behaviour.
D. The attachment figure provides excessive physical contact.
E. The attachment figure shows inconsistent responses.

1.12 Separation during the critical period (Bowlby):
A. Takes place before the age of 3 months.
B. Initially produces despair.
C. Ultimately produces detachment.
D. When prolonged is associated with dwarfed growth.
E. When sustained is associated with developmental language delay.

1.9

A. False – The Hawthorne effect is when presence of the interviewer alters the situation and influences the responses. The description is that of the Halo effect.

B. True.

C. False – In fact the opposite: tendency to select extremes.

D. False – The Halo effect describes answer selection to fit with other responses. The description is that of social acceptability error.

E. False – In Logical error there is a logical link in rating the items. The selection of extremes is described as a leniency error.

1.10

A. False – IQ = (mental age/chronological age) 100.

B. True – Component intelligence is that used for executive tasks and experiential intelligence is that used for routine tasks that have already been learnt/mastered.

C. True.

D. False – Measured intelligence increases up to 16 years of age after which it plateaus till 25 years of age. There is then a gradual decline.

E. True.

1.11

A. False – The child displays muted clinginess.

B. True.

C. True – Avoidant attachment may lead to aggressive behaviour later in life.

D. False – The attachment figure provides less physical contact.

E. False – The attachment figure shows less sensitivity.

1.12

A. False – The critical period is ages 6 months to 3 years (Bowlby).

B. False – Initially produces protest and then despair.

C. True – This follows despair.

D. True – Prolonged separation (maternal deprivation) is also associated with attention-seeking and aggressive behaviour.

E. True.

1.13 Social class:
  A. Is usually defined according to fixed social parameters.
  B. As described by the Registrar General's classification includes unskilled, skilled and highly skilled categories.
  C. In Britain is based primarily on occupation.
  D. Is unrelated to smoking.
  E. Is not ascribed to those that are unemployed.

1.14 Sigmund Freud published the following:
  A. *The Interpretation of Dreams.*
  B. *The Ego and the Id.*
  C. *The Ego and the Mechanisms of Defence.*
  D. *Childhood and Society.*
  E. *Three Essays on the Theory of Sexuality.*

1.15 Carl Gustav Jung:
  A. Developed transactional analysis.
  B. In addition to the personal unconscious proposed the objective psyche.
  C. Described networks of ideas and thoughts that he called complexes.
  D. Believed in the concept of individuation.
  E. Described personalities as extroverted and introverted.

1.13

A. False – The parameters (money, occupation, education) are relatively stable but not fixed and hence there is mobility between the various classes.
B. False – Semi-skilled category (Class IV). There is no highly skilled category.
C. True – Occupation of the head of the household.
D. False – Disease-promoting behaviours are more common in lower social classes.
E. False – Unemployed = Class O.

Note: Registrar General's Classification of social class – Professional, intermediate, skilled, semi-skilled, unskilled, unemployed (I, II, III, IV, V, O).

1.14

A. True – Published in 1900.
B. True – Published in 1923.
C. False – Published by his daughter Anna Freud.
D. False – Published by Erik Erikson in 1950.
E. True.

1.15

A. False – Jung is recognized as the founder of analytical psychology. Eric Berne developed transactional analysis.
B. True – This is more commonly known as the collective unconscious.
C. True – These ideas and thoughts are linked through commonality of emotions and feelings. They surround archetypes and evolve out of archetype–experience interactions.
D. True – This was the ultimate goal in which the growth of an individual's personality leads to self-realization and understanding.
E. True – Jung disagreed with Freud and placed less emphasis on the sexual role of the libido. Instead he viewed the libido as stemming from all psychic and life energy. He therefore described personality organization as outwardly focused (outwardly directed libido: extroversion) and inwardly focused (inwardly directed libido: introversion).

1.16 Kleinian theory:
- A. Differs from Freudian theory in that there is no concept of an ego.
- B. Suggests that the paranoid–schizoid position develops in the third year of life.
- C. Describes the depressive position as arising out of persecutory anxiety.
- D. Considers introjection and projection to be the primary defence mechanisms in operation in the first few months of life.
- E. Proposes that infants are capable of object relations.

1.17 The following are correctly paired:
- A. Jacob Moreno and psychodrama.
- B. Wilfred Bion and self-actualization.
- C. Egas Moniz and psychosurgery.
- D. Heinz Kohut and self-psychology.
- E. Adolf Meyer and primal anxiety.

1.18 Descriptions of thought disorder proposed by Schneider include:
- A. Substitution.
- B. Tangentiality.
- C. Schizophasia.
- D. Omission.
- E. Interpenetration.

1.16

A. False – In fact the ego is thought to develop in the first year of life.
B. False – This takes place in the infant year.
C. False – Persecutory anxiety like aggression are associated with the development of the paranoid–schizoid position.
D. True – Splitting is also an important defence mechanism: splitting into good and bad elements.
E. True – That they are able to internalize experiences of the external world.

1.17

A. True.
B. False – Wilfred Bion applied the ideas of psychoanalysis to groups and described the three basic assumptions: pairing, fight–flight and dependency. Psychodrama is associated with Jacob Moreno.
C. True – and Almeida Lima.
D. True.
E. False – Adolf Meyer founded psychobiology. He had a holistic approach, aiming to understand people and their illnesses in the simplest terms possible.

1.18

A. True – A principal thought or idea is replaced by a subsidiary thought or idea.
B. False – Oblique verbal response that only glances at gist.
C. False – Word salad: words are jumbled to the extent that they are difficult to understand.
D. True – Senseless omission of a segment of thought.
E. False – Described by Cameron.

Note: Others include fusion, derailment, desultory thinking, drivelling.

1.19 The following terms are correctly described:
   A. Akataphasia: the verbal component of catatonia.
   B. Prolixity: flight of ideas in which the train of thought eventually returns to its original track.
   C. Echolalia: repetition of another individual's speech using own words or phrases.
   D. Dysphonia: akin to cacophony, the perception of discordant sound.
   E. Stock word: one that is used repeatedly.

1.20 Cranial nerves:
   A. Olfactory nerve tertiary neurones pass through the cribriform plate.
   B. Obstructive hydrocephalus is a cause of anosmia.
   C. The lateral geniculate body is not involved in the accommodation reflex.
   D. The Holmes–Adie pupil is small (constricted).
   E. The Edinger Westphal nucleus provides parasympathetic innervation to the constrictor pupillae.

1.21 Neurological complications of alcohol abuse include:
   A. Granulovacuolar degeneration.
   B. Mammillary body haemorrhage.
   C. Cerebellar degeneration.
   D. Sclerotic plaques.
   E. Corpus callosum degeneration.

1.19

A. False – Used by Kraepelin to describe thought disorder manifest in speech.
B. True.
C. False – This is echologia. In echolalia the imitation and repetition of speech is exact.
D. False – Impaired ability to vocalize.
E. False – Can be used repeatedly, however, it refers to a word that is used in a peculiar manner to have more than its usual significance or meaning.

1.20

A. False – Primary neurones from nasal mucosa receptors pass through the cribriform plate.
B. True – Although this is a relatively rare cause of anosmia.
C. False – It is involved in accommodation but not in the light reflex.
D. False – It is large (dilated).
E. True – Also to the ciliary muscles.

1.21

A. False.
B. True.
C. True.
D. False.
E. True – (Marchiafava–Bignami syndrome).

Note: Other neurological complications/effects of alcohol misuse include seizures, peripheral neuropathy, optic atrophy and central pontine myelinolysis.

1.22 Saccades (saccadic eye movements):
  A. Are rapid, purposeful, conjugate eye movements.
  B. Are impaired by frontal lobe lesions.
  C. Are abnormal in schizophrenia.
  D. Are abnormal in Wernicke–Korsakoff syndrome.
  E. When abnormal, are a reliable, early sign of Huntingdon's disease.

1.23 Features of frontal lobe lesions include:
  A. Utilization behaviour.
  B. Palmo-mental reflex.
  C. Perseveration.
  D. Expressive aphasia.
  E. Apathy.

1.22

A. True – Saccades are characterized by their speed. The eyes move rapidly but smoothly towards any object that appears in the periphery of the visual field.

B. True – Frontal lobe lesions impair saccades and occipital, parietal and brainstem lesions impair pursuit movements. However, extensive cerebral lesions which involve the supranuclear gaze centres impair both pursuit and saccadic eye movement.

C. True.

D. False.

E. True – Abnormal saccades are not specific and simply indicate that there is some underlying biological abnormality.

1.23

A. True – An example of this inappropriate behaviour – the patient upon noticing a syringe in the doctor's surgery attempts to use it.

B. True – Wartenberg's reflex. Gentle scratching of the thenar eminence produces contraction of the ipsilateral mentalis muscle which results in dimpling of the chin.

C. True – Individual continues to perform a particular action beyond its relevance.

D. True – Indicates involvement of Broca's area (Brodmann's areas 44 and 45) within frontal operculum on dominant side.

E. True – Other changes include irritability, impairment of social drive and initiative, and disruptive and socially inappropriate behaviour.

1.24 The following are features of upper motor neurone lesions:
   A. Fasciculation.
   B. Clonus.
   C. Absent cremasteric reflex.
   D. Wasting.
   E. Weakness and clumsiness.

1.25 Recognized pathological features of Pick's disease cerebral tissue include:
   A. Lewy bodies.
   B. Balloon cells.
   C. Marked parieto-occipital atrophy.
   D. Knife-blade gyri.
   E. Fibrous gliosis.

1.26 Recognized pathological features of Creutzfeldt–Jakob disease cerebral tissue include:
   A. Marked brain atrophy.
   B. Proliferation of inflammatory cells.
   C. Cortical grey matter status spongiosus.
   D. Intraneuronal prion protein.
   E. Astrocyte proliferation.

1.24

A. False – This is the involuntary, spontaneous contraction of groups of muscle fibres that form part of a motor unit. It is seen in lower motor neurone lesions, especially those affecting anterior horn cells (e.g. motor neurone disease).

B. True – Also have spasticity and increased tendon reflexes.

C. True – This is a superficial reflex like the abdominal reflex. These are absent in pyramidal lesions.

D. False – Wasting occurs in lower motor neurone lesions except with neuropraxia (consequence of nerve compression).

E. True – There is a pyramidal pattern of weakness accompanied by clumsiness in which there is a loss of the fine dextrous movements of the digits of the hand.

1.25

A. False – Lewy bodies, plaques and neurofibrillary tangles are absent.

B. True – Another name for Pick cells. Swollen cortical pyramidal cells.

C. False – Characteristically find marked asymmetrical fronto-temporal atrophy.

D. True – Gyri take on brownish appearance with spongiform change.

E. True – There is also marked neuronal loss from cortex, basal ganglia, substantia nigra and locus coeruleus and astrocyte proliferation.

1.26

A. False – Brain atrophy is minimal.

B. False – Even though the disease is 'infective' there is an absence of inflammation.

C. True – This distinctive microscopic sponge-like appearance is also seen in the thalamus, basal ganglia and motor nuclei.

D. True – This protease-resistant prion protein accumulates in neurones and forms plaques.

E. True.

1.27 Neuroglia:
A. Outnumber neurones 2:1.
B. Make up 10% of normal brain volume.
C. Are present in the retina.
D. Are non-conducting.
E. Continually undergo mitosis.

1.28 CNS axons:
A. Are myelinated by Schwann cells.
B. Possess an initial segment devoid of intracellular inclusions such as Nissl granules.
C. Like dendrites contain both neurofilaments and micro-tubules.
D. Conduct away from the perikaryon and rarely undergo arborization.
E. Contain Tau protein.

1.29 Clinical features of Parkinson's disease include:
A. Ataxic gait.
B. Depression.
C. Bradyphrenia.
D. Macrographia.
E. Seborrhoea.

1.27

   A.   False – Neuroglia outnumber neurones 10:1.

   B.   False – Neuroglia make up 50% of normal brain volume.

   C.   True – Called Muller cells.

   D.   True.

   E.   True.

Note: Neuroglia include astrocytes, oligodendrocytes, microglia, ependyma, Muller cells (retina), pituicytes (posterior pituitary) and Bergman cells (cerebellum).

1.28

   A.   False – Peripheral nerves are myelinated by Schwann cells. CNS myelination is carried out by oligodendrocytes.

   B.   True – The axonal initial segment stems from the neuronal soma as the axon hillock which is also devoid of intracellular inclusions such as Nissl granules (ribosomes).

   C.   True – N.B. Axons contain more neurofilaments than microtubules and the reverse is true for dendrites.

   D.   True.

   E.   True – This is specific to axons as opposed to dendrites.

1.29

   A.   False – Classically patients have a shuffling, festinant gait.

   B.   True – 50% of patients. Suicide rate is low and guilt is less common.

   C.   True – Other cognitive deficits include poor recent memory and difficulty with abstract reasoning.

   D.   False – Micrographia (small handwriting).

   E.   True – Sialorrhoea (excessive salivation) and seborrhoea (greasy skin) are common findings.

1.30 Characteristic clinical features of Wilson's disease include:
A. Choreoathetosis.
B. Bilateral ptosis.
C. Jaundice.
D. Dysarthria.
E. Flaccid paralysis.

1.31 Stage 2 non-REM sleep:
A. Forms 50% of total sleep time.
B. Is characterized by K complexes and sleep spindles on EEG.
C. Usually precedes REM sleep.
D. Increases cerebral blood flow.
E. Features myoclonic jerks.

1.32 Axon myelination:
A. Is performed by Schwann cells in the peripheral nervous system.
B. Results in saltatory conduction.
C. Is complete prior to birth.
D. Supports regeneration of damaged peripheral nerves.
E. Precedes neuronal growth.

1.30

A. True – Often have a wide flapping tremor of the arms sometimes described as a bat-wing or wing-beating tremor.
B. False – Seen in myaesthenia gravis.
C. True – Copper deposition in the liver produces hepatitis, hepatosplenomegaly and cirrhosis.
D. True – Also experience dysphagia.
E. False – Instead often experience rigidity.

1.31

A. True – 75% of sleep is spent in non-REM sleep and more than two-thirds of this consists of stage 2 sleep.
B. True.
C. True – REM sleep is usually entered after about 90 minutes of sleep, from stage 2 of non-REM sleep.
D. False – Parasympathetic activity is predominant in non-REM sleep. Cerebral blood flow is diminished.
E. False – These occur during REM sleep.

1.32

A. True – In the central nervous system oligodendrocytes perform the same function.
B. True – Between each segment of myelination there are segments of unmyelinated axon. These are called nodes of Ranvier and action potentials effectively jump from one node to the next. This is called saltatory conduction.
C. False – Myelination begins at the start of the second trimester and continues after birth. It is usually completed within the first year of life.
D. True – Peripheral nerve degeneration, for example due to trauma, results in phagocytic resorption of neuronal elements. However, the myelin tube remains and this aids regeneration and growth of the regenerating tip.
E. False – Myelin segments grow along with the nerve fibres.

1.33 Acetylcholine:
A. Is synthesized from choline and coenzyme A.
B. Is stored in intraneuronal vesicles.
C. Is inactivated by the glycoprotein acetylcholinesterase.
D. Degradation produces choline and acetic acid.
E. Synthesis is inhibited by edrophonium.

1.34 Tyrosine hydroxylase:
A. Is the rate-limiting enzyme in catecholamine synthesis.
B. Is inhibited by Fe^{2+} ions.
C. Is inhibited by α-methyl-para-tyrosine.
D. Is inhibited by catecholamines.
E. Is present in all sympathetically innervated tissues.

1.35 Catecholamines:
A. Are transported into secretory vesicles against an electrochemical gradient.
B. Include dopamine and serotonin.
C. Are metabolized by monoamine oxidase and catechol-*O*-methyltransferase.
D. Are released at synapses by methylphenidate.
E. Undergo active synaptic re-uptake that can be inhibited by oubain.

1.33

A. False – It is synthesized from choline and acetyl CoA in a single reaction catalysed by choline acetyl-transferase.

B. True – These vesicles originate in the cell body and are transported to the nerve terminals. After acetylcholine release the vesicles are re-cycled.

C. True – Acetylcholinesterase is found in both brain and muscle and catalyses the degradation of acetylcholine to produce choline and acetic acid.

D. True.

E. False – Acetylcholine synthesis can be inhibited by hemicholinium-3 and triethylcholine. Edrophonium is a competitive anticholinesterase that is used to diagnose Myaesthenia Gravis.

1.34

A. True.

B. False – Tyrosine hydroxylase requires Fe^{2+}, molecular oxygen and tetrahydropteridine cofactor. It is stereo-specific and oxidizes only L-tyrosine.

C. True – Four groups of tyrosine hydroxylase inhibitors: catechol derivatives, tropolones, amino acid analogues and selective iron chelators.

D. True – End-product inhibition.

E. True – Especially adrenal medulla and brain.

1.35

A. False – An electrical potential and intra-vesicular pH of between 5 and 6 (created by active proton translocation) favours the movement of catecholamines into vesicles.

B. False – Dopamine, noradrenaline and adrenaline are catecholamines. Serotonin is an indolealkylamine.

C. True.

D. True – Amphetamine also leads to synaptic release of catecholamines.

E. True – Synaptic uptake is an active process and this is inhibited by oubain.

1.36 L-Tryptophan:
  A. Is an acidic amino acid.
  B. Adjunctive therapy is used in the treatment of resistant depression.
  C. Causes drowsiness.
  D. Oxidation produces serotonin.
  E. Plasma levels are largely determined by diet.

1.37 The following drugs are teratogenic:
  A. Warfarin.
  B. Heparin.
  C. Paracetamol.
  D. Fluoxetine.
  E. Primidone.

1.36

A. False – Aspartate and glutamate are acidic amino acids. Tryptophan is a non-polar (neutral amino acid).
B. True – Its use is limited. Its previous association with eosinophilia–myalgia syndrome necessitates registration and close supervision.
C. True – Can be quite marked..
D. False – Hydroxylation by tryptophan hydroxylase produces serotonin.
E. True – Consequently plasma levels fluctuate and can be experimentally lowered to induce depressed mood.

1.37

A. True – Warfarin freely crosses the placenta and a foetal warfarin syndrome (epiphyseal stippling, nasal hypoplasia) has been described. Risk from first trimester exposure is about 5%.
B. False – Heparin does not cross the placenta. It is not teratogenic, however, it is associated with osteoporosis.
C. False – Paracetamol is not known to be harmful during pregnancy.
D. False – The use of SSRIs, including fluoxetine, is only advised if any potential benefit outweighs possible risks. However, thus far, there is no evidence of teratogenicity.
E. True – Primidone is metabolized to phenobarbitone. It is teratogenic.

Note: During the first trimester of pregnancy, especially weeks 3–11, drugs that cross the placenta may produce congenital malformations (teratogenesis).

1.38 Chlorpromazine:
  A. Interacts with anterior pituitary lobe mammotroph D2 receptors.
  B. Can be administered per rectum in the form of suppositories.
  C. Metabolism yields more than 100 metabolites.
  D. Indications include the induction of hyperthermia.
  E. 100 mg is equivalent to approximately 20 mg of haloperidol (oral doses).

1.39 Clozapine:
  A. Has greater antagonist activity at D1 receptors than at D2 receptors.
  B. Is absorbed relatively slowly from the gastrointestinal tract and reaches peak plasma levels within 24–48 hours.
  C. Is a dibenzodiazepine.
  D. Causes agranulocytosis in approximately 8–11% of patients.
  E. Is occasionally useful in the treatment of toxic psychoses.

1.38

  A. True – Tuberoinfundibular dopamine acts on these receptors to inhibit prolactin release. Chlorpromazine blockade of these receptors leads to hyperprolactinaemia.
  B. True – Chlorpromazine can also be given orally as tablets, solution or syrup and can also be given by deep intramuscular injection.
  C. True – Some of these metabolites are active.
  D. False – Chlorpromazine is indicated in schizophrenia and other psychoses, mania, violent behaviour and the short-term management of severe anxiety. It is also used to treat intractable hiccups and in the induction of *hypo*thermia.
  E. False – An oral dose of 100 mg chlorpromazine is approximately equivalent to 2–3 mg of haloperidol.

1.39

  A. True – It also acts at $5HT_2$, α_1 and α_2, cholinergic and histaminergic receptors.
  B. False – It is rapidly absorbed from the gastrointestinal tract and reaches peak plasma levels within 1–4 hours. It is metabolized completely with a half-life of about 16 hours.
  C. True – Clozapine is a dibenzodiazepine.
  D. False – It does cause agranulocytosis but only in about 3% of patients. This compares with 0.5% of patients treated with typical antipsychotics.
  E. False – It is contra-indicated in the treatment of alcoholic and toxic psychoses.

Note: Clozapine also causes sedation, sialorrhoea and seizures. Its use requires registration with the Clozaril Patient Monitoring Service.

1.40 Priapism is a side-effect of the following:
A. Clozapine.
B. Paracetamol.
C. Risperidone.
D. Alprostadil.
E. Trazodone.

1.41 The following statements about Mendelian Inheritance are correct:
A. It does not apply to single gene defects.
B. Mendel's first Law is also known as the law of uniformity.
C. Autosomal dominant inheritance gives the appearance of horizontal transmission.
D. X-linked recessive inheritance results in male carriers.
E. There is an increased incidence of parental consanguinity in autosomal recessive inheritance.

1.42 Down's syndrome:
A. Is responsible for 90% of those with mental retardation and IQ < 50.
B. Occurs in approximately 1 in 20 000 births.
C. Arises most often because of translocation of genetic material between chromosome 21 and another.
D. Recurrence is more likely with non-disjunction than translocation.
E. Is associated with a marked reduction in P300 latency.

1.43 Cri-du-chat syndrome:
A. Is associated with hypotonia.
B. Is equally common in males and females.
C. Arises because of a deletion.
D. Results in hypertelorism.
E. Occurs in 1 in 50 000 births.

1.40

A. True.
B. False.
C. True.
D. True – Used as a diagnostic test and as a treatment for erectile dysfunction.
E. True.

Note: Priapism requires urgent treatment (within 6 hours) and involves initially penile aspiration. If this is unsuccessful intracavernosal injections of phenylephrine, adrenaline or metaraminol (α adrenoceptor sympathomimetics) can be cautiously attempted before resorting to surgical means.

1.41

A. False – It applies to single gene defects (deletions, insertions, inversions).
B. False – Mendel's first law is the law of segregation and the second law is the law of independent assortment.
C. False – The phenotypic trait is evident in every generation and so the appearance is that of vertical transmission.
D. False – All males with the affected allele manifest the disorder whereas females can be carriers if heterozygous.
E. True.

1.42

A. False – Significantly high but only one-third.
B. False – Overall incidence is 1:660 live births.
C. False – Most common cause (95% of cases) is non-disjunction.
D. False – Recurrence is more likely with translocation. With non-disjunction risk is approximately 1%.
E. False – It is associated with a marked increase in P300 latency.

1.43

A. False – It is associated with spasticity.
B. False – More common in females.
C. True – Deletion on short arm chromosome 5.
D. True – And an alert expression.
E. True.

1.44 The following are genetic deletion defects:
A. Retinoblastoma.
B. Patau's syndrome.
C. Prader–Willi syndrome.
D. Wilm's tumour.
E. Rett's disorder.

1.45 The following are gut–brain neuropeptides:
A. Somatotropin.
B. Substance P.
C. Melatonin.
D. Somatostatin.
E. Neurotensin.

1.46 As compared to classic neurotransmitters, peptide neurotransmitters:
A. Have high receptor affinity.
B. Have low receptor potency.
C. Are effective at smaller concentrations.
D. Undergo less neuronal re-uptake.
E. Are synthesized more quickly.

1.44

   A.   True – Deletion (chromosome 13).

   B.   False – Trisomy 13.

   C.   True – Deletion (chromosome 15).

   D.   True – Deletion (chromosome 11).

   E.   False – X-linked dominant disorder. Affects females only.

1.45

   A.   False – This is another name for growth hormone which is a 190 amino acid protein released from the anterior pituitary.

   B.   True – It is an 11 amino acid gut peptide discovered in 1931. It is present in the brain (substantia nigra, cerebral cortex, hypothalamus, amygdala, striatum) and spinal cord. It is involved in pathways concerning pain and movement.

   C.   False – Melatonin is not a peptide and is synthesized in the pineal gland from serotonin.

   D.   True – It is a 14 amino acid peptide that is found in the Islets of Langerhans. It is also found in the striatum, amygdala and cerebral cortex.

   E.   True – It is a 13 amino acid peptide found in the spinal cord (substantia gelatinosa), hypothalamus, pituitary, amygdala, septum, nucleus accumbens and brain stem.

1.46

   A.   False – Peptide neurotransmitters have relatively low receptor affinity but relatively high receptor potency.

   B.   False.

   C.   True – Effective at picomolar concentrations as compared to micromolar/nanomolar concentrations.

   D.   True – Neuronal re-uptake of peptide neurotransmitters is insignificant.

   E.   False – Peptide neurotransmitters are synthesized as pre-pro-peptides that undergo enzymatic conversion in the soma. The process is relatively slow.

1.47 The following are derived from pro-opiomelanocortin (POMC):
A. Dynorphin.
B. Met-enkephalin.
C. β-endorphin.
D. Corticotrophin-releasing hormone (CRH).
E. Melatonin.

1.48 In statistics:
A. The power of a test is the probability that the null hypothesis will be correctly rejected.
B. A one-tailed test is used if differences are hypothesized to occur in only one direction.
C. A type I error is that of incorrectly rejecting the alternative hypothesis.
D. Parametric tests can be applied as long as one of the variables is measured on an interval or ratio scale.
E. The variance is a measure of central tendency.

1.49 For values 1, 4, 1, 3, 1:
A. The arithmetic mean is 2
B. The mode is 1
C. The median is 2
D. The geometric mean is $^5\sqrt{12}$
E. The range is 5

1.50 Computerized tomography (CT):
A. Uses X-ray photons.
B. Measures proton density.
C. Has an in-slice resolution of $< 1 \mu$m.
D. Is better at detecting calcified brain lesions than magnetic resonance imaging.
E. On a CT image cerebrospinal fluid appears white.

1.47

A. False – Dynorphin is derived from prodynorphin.
B. False – Met-enkephalin and leu-enkephalin are both derived from proenkephalins.
C. True – POMC also contains the amino acid sequences for β-lipotrophin, melanocyte-stimulating hormone and ACTH.
D. False – CRH is a hypothalamic-releasing hormone that acts on the anterior pituitary.
E. False – Melatonin is synthesized from serotonin in the pineal gland.

1.48

A. True – The null hypothesis is false and is recognized as such.
B. True.
C. False – This is a type II error, i.e. wrongly concluding that there are no differences.
D. True.
E. False – It is a measure of dispersion.

1.49

A. True – Sum of the magnitude of the items divided by the number of items.
B. True – The most frequent item.
C. False – The median is the middle value when the values are ranked in order. 1, 1, **1**, 3, 4. The answer is 1.
D. True – For numbers 1 to n it is the nth root of the product of the numbers.
E. False – It is the difference between the highest and lowest values. The answer is 3.

1.50

A. True – Based on X-ray attenuation.
B. False – Measures tissue density.
C. False – In-slice resolution is < 1 mm.
D. True.
E. False – It appears black.

Paper 2

2.1 In respondent learning:
A. Incubation refers to the delay in learning.
B. Extinction is the disappearance of the learned response.
C. The optimal acquisition stage is 0.5 s.
D. Discrimination is diminished by differential reinforcement.
E. Stimulus generalization increases in proportion to stimulus novelty.

2.2 Effective models for observational learning:
A. Are of similar age.
B. Have high status.
C. Possess social power.
D. Are competent.
E. Are of the opposite sex.

2.3 Development of vision; the following are correct:
A. At birth the infant's visual focus is fixed at a distance of 2 m.
B. Accurate acuity is usually achieved in the first month of life.
C. An infant less than 6 months old cannot differentiate complex stimuli such as human faces.
D. Four month old infants are able to accommodate.
E. Colour vision is present at birth.

2.1

    A.   False – Incubation describes the increase in the strength of the conditioned response that follows repeated brief exposure to the conditioned stimulus.

    B.   True – When the conditioned stimulus is repeatedly presented without the unconditioned stimulus the conditioned response gradually disappears.

    C.   False – The acquisition stage is the period of association between the unconditioned stimulus and the conditioned stimulus. It is selective and variable.

    D.   False – Discrimination is the ability to recognize and respond to the differences between similar stimuli and can be produced by differential reinforcement.

    E.   False – It decreases in proportion to the novelty of the new stimulus.

2.2

    A.   True – Similarity is an important feature.

    B.   True.

    C.   True.

    D.   True.

    E.   False – Again similarity enhances effectiveness and similarity with observer is important.

2.3

    A.   False – It is fixed but at a distance of 0.2 m.

    B.   False – 6:6 vision is not achieved until almost 6 months old.

    C.   False – Able to differentiate faces by end of first month.

    D.   True.

    E.   False – Develops usually by age of 4 months.

Note: Development of vision is dependent on interaction with the environment.

2.4 Memory retrieval:
A. Recency effect is because these items undergo most consolidation.
B. Long-term memory retrieval is facilitated by reproducing original emotional context.
C. Memory is recalled from long-term memory to sensory memory.
D. The primacy effect occurs because of anxiety.
E. Implicit retrieval involves no conscious recollection or temporal awareness.

2.5 Attitudes:
A. Serve an instrumental function.
B. The affective component, that is the feelings towards the attitude object, can be easily changed.
C. Tend to predict behaviour best when based on the subject's personal experience.
D. Are thought to comprise three independent components.
E. Can be assessed by sociometry.

2.6 In Festinger's cognitive dissonance theory increased dissonance occurs when:
A. Pressure to comply is high.
B. There is an awareness of personal responsibility for any consequences.
C. Perceived choice is low.
D. Consequences of alternative behaviour are pleasurable.
E. Behaviour can be altered.

2.7 Persuasive communicators:
A. Possess credibility.
B. Have a vested interest in the message.
C. Are recognized opinion leaders.
D. Are very different to recipients of message.
E. Use non-verbal cues.

2.4

   A. False – It is because these items are still within short-term memory.

   B. True – State-dependent learning.

   C. False – From long-term memory to short-term memory.

   D. False – It occurs because the initial items receive most consolidation.

   E. True.

2.5

   A. True.

   B. False – This component is most resistant to change.

   C. True – Also when consistent and strong and related specifically to the predicted behaviour.

   D. False – The three components, affective, behavioural and cognitive, are thought to influence each other.

   E. True – Subjects in groups nominate preferred partners and create sociograms which identify sub-groups.

2.6

   A. False – The opposite is true, i.e. pressure to comply is low.

   B. True.

   C. False – When perceived choice is high.

   D. False – When consequences of alternative behaviour are anticipated to be unpleasant.

   E. False – Altering behaviour can help to reduce dissonance-associated anxiety/tension.

2.7

   A. True – Possess expertise.

   B. False – Have genuine motivation.

   C. True.

   D. False – Are similar and therefore recipients are able to identify with communicator.

   E. True.

Note: Other important aspects of persuasive communicators are that they be likeable and attractive.

2.8 Thurstone's proposed primary mental abilities include:
  A. Aptitude.
  B. Reasoning.
  C. Perceptual speed.
  D. Colour.
  E. Memory.

2.9 The Wechsler Adult Intelligence Scale (WAIS):
  A. Is a component of the Halstead Reitan Neuropsychological Battery (HRNB).
  B. Digit symbol sub-test provides a score towards verbal IQ.
  C. Consists of more verbal sub-tests than performance sub-tests.
  D. Is inappropriate for individuals less than 18 years of age.
  E. Is also known as the Wechsler Memory Scale.

2.10 The following statements concerning validity are correct:
  A. Face validity: extent to which all aspects of the subject matter are assessed.
  B. Convergent validity: a form of criterion validity.
  C. Divergent validity: the degree to which a measure discriminates that being assessed from unrelated measures.
  D. Concurrent validity: the extent to which the criterion validity of a measure is retained when applied to a new set of subjects.
  E. Predictive validity: ability to predict outcome as measured now and in the future or on another scale.

2.11 In dysfunctional families:
  A. Parents are over-involved and stifle the child's individuality.
  B. Parents are under-involved.
  C. Members of the family are excessively close.
  D. Communication problems are rare.
  E. Triangulation occurs.

2.8

A. False – Aptitude is not described and refers to potential ability.
B. True – Others include, number, word fluency, verbal comprehension and space.
C. True.
D. False.
E. True.

2.9

A. True – The HRNB is used for diagnosing brain damage and comprises 11 components, one of which is the WAIS.
B. False – Digit symbol is a performance sub-test which involves symbol substitution. Its scaled score contributes towards an overall performance IQ.
C. True – There are six sub-tests which assess verbal skills and five that assess performance (non-verbal skills).
D. False – It is designed for those aged 16 years and over. Below this age (5–15 years) the Wechsler Intelligence Scale for Children (WISC) can be used.
E. False – This is a separate assessment scale which predominantly tests learning and short-term memory.

2.10

A. False – This describes content validity. Face validity: whether the intended characteristic appears to be measured.
B. False – It is a form of construct validity.
C. True.
D. False – This describes cross-validity. Concurrent validity is the comparison of simultaneous measures involving reference to an external measure.
E. True.

2.11

A. True – This is termed enmeshment.
B. True – Termed rejection this results in loneliness.
C. True – This is an aspect of enmeshment.
D. False – Communication problems are very common.
E. True – This refers to the development of exclusive relationships.

2.12 The following are equally likely sequelae of both physical and sexual abuse:
A. Depression.
B. Eating disorders.
C. Dissociation.
D. Borderline personality disorder.
E. Child molestation.

2.13 The Black Report (1980):
A. Principally examined immigrant status and social class.
B. Reported that those from social class V were 10 times as likely to die as those from social class I.
C. Identified a higher neonatal mortality in those from social class V as compared with those from social class I.
D. Identified high levels of unemployment in Indians of Kenyan origin as compared with Afro-Caribbeans.
E. Noted an increased rate of most diseases in the lower social classes.

2.14 In Karl Abraham's expansion of Freud's theory of psychosexual development:
A. The genital phase begins at 7 years of age.
B. The oral phase is split into receptive and retentive phases.
C. The anal phase includes an expulsive phase.
D. The phallic phase involves aggression towards the opposite sex parent.
E. The period of latency occurs at the same time as Piaget's concrete operational stage.

2.15 Jung described the following psychological functions as the basic operations of the mind:
A. Dreaming.
B. Sensation.
C. Feeling.
D. Intuition.
E. Thinking.

2.12

A. True – Both forms of abuse diminish the affected individual's self-esteem.
B. False – This is more likely to follow sexual abuse than physical abuse.
C. True.
D. True – There is also a predisposition to self-harm.
E. False – This is more likely to follow sexual abuse than physical abuse.

2.13

A. False – It examined health in relation to social class.
B. False – The likelihood is doubled, i.e. twice as likely to die prior to retirement.
C. True.
D. False.
E. True.

2.14

A. False – The genital phase begins with the onset of puberty at around 12 years of age.
B. False – It is split into an early sucking stage and a later biting stage referred to as receptive and sadistic phases, respectively.
C. True – It also includes a retentive phase.
D. False – Aggression is directed towards the same sex parent.
E. True – Approximately 6–12 years of age.

2.15

A. False.
B. True – Acquisition of information.
C. True – The realization of experiences, e.g. emotion.
D. True – This refers to perception via unconscious mechanisms and processes.
E. True – Thought, reason, logic.

Note: These four basic mental operations are combined with the two attitudes (introversion and extroversion) to create eight psychological types.

2.16 Alfred Adler:
- A. Founded analytical psychology.
- B. Developed the concept of organ inferiority.
- C. Proposed an interpersonal theory of personality.
- D. Introduced the term masculine protest.
- E. Encouraged individuals to direct their own fate and gain a sense of dignity and worth.

2.17 The following terms are described correctly:
- A. Vorbeirden: the interweaving of two differing streams of thought (fusion).
- B. Entgleisen: inexplicable, unanticipated abrupt cessation of thought.
- C. Paragrammatism: comprehensible phrases which collectively fail to make sense or convey any meaning.
- D. Asyndesis: a principal thought or idea is replaced by a subsidiary thought or idea.
- E. Perseveration: persistence of cued speech beyond its relevance.

2.18 The following definitions are correct:
- A. Alexithymia: the inability to verbally express one's emotions.
- B. Moria: morbid preoccupation with death.
- C. Sthenic affects: sadness, grief and shame.
- D. Verstimmung: moodiness, an ill-humoured mood state usually with depressive symptomatology.
- E. Dysphoria: chronic state of low mood, usually of insidious onset and lasting at least 2 years.

2.19 Cranial nerves:
- A. Oculomotor nerve damage results in nasal deviation of the eyeball.
- B. The trochlear nerve supplies the inferior oblique.
- C. Abducens nerve palsy is rare.
- D. The trigeminal nerve motor component supplies the pterygoid muscles.
- E. The efferent limb of the corneal reflex is transmitted in the ophthalmic nerve.

2.16

A. False – Jung developed analytical psychology. Adler developed individual psychology.
B. True.
C. False – Harry Stack Sullivan proposed this, in which interpersonal experiences form the basis of personality development.
D. True – This is an individual's attempt to escape a submissive feminine role.
E. True – Instead of being subject to unconscious drives. Emphasized social co-operation and creativity.

2.17

A. False – Fusion is a kind of thought disorder described by Schneider. Vorbeirden is talking past the point.
B. False – This describes thought block (entgleiten). Entgleisen is derailment in which the main theme is displaced by intrusion of subsidiary themes and these too then undergo displacement.
C. True.
D. False – Asyndesis: a lack of sufficient connections between successive elements of thought.
E. True.

2.18

A. True.
B. False – Fatuous affect also termed Witzelsucht describes apathy and silliness combined with general indifference.
C. False – These are asthenic affects. Sthenic affects include hate, anger, rage and joy.
D. True.
E. False – This describes dysthymia. Dysphoria is simply an unpleasant mood.

2.19

A. False – Eyeball is directed 'down and out'.
B. False – Superior oblique.
C. False – It is the commonest cranial nerve palsy.
D. True – Also the masseters – muscles of mastication.
E. False – This is the afferent limb. Efferent limb to orbicularis oris effects bilateral blink and is transmitted in facial nerve.

Paper 2

2.20 Diplopia:
A. When monocular, usually persists in all directions of gaze.
B. When binocular, is abolished by covering either eye.
C. Is caused by supranuclear lesions.
D. Develops with congenital ocular muscle weakness (strabismus).
E. Is caused by brainstem infarction.

2.21 The following cause the visual field defects described:
A. Craniopharyngioma – tunnel vision.
B. Cerebral infarction – homonymous hemianopia.
C. Optic neuritis – monocular central scotoma.
D. Interruption of Meyer's loop – superior quadrantanopia.
E. Pituitary adenoma – bitemporal hemianopia.

2.22 First-order dorsal column axons:
A. Carry sensory information from Ruffini's endings.
B. Subserving pressure sensation terminate in the intralaminar nuclei of the thalamus.
C. Subserving vibration sensation terminate in the gracile and cuneate nuclei.
D. Decussate in the medial lemniscus.
E. Carry sensory information from Merkel's disks.

2.20

A. True – Monocular diplopia is usually the result of ocular abnormalities (retinal tear, lens dislocation). Diplopia occurs when the normal eye is covered.
B. True – Usually occurs because of neurological injuries and manifests only in specific directions of gaze.
C. False – Supranuclear lesions result in conjugate palsies.
D. False – In these cases the brain suppresses the image from the weaker eye and can result in blindness.
E. True – Other causes include weakness of the extraocular muscles (e.g. myaesthenia gravis), and third and sixth cranial nerve injury.

2.21

A. False – Lesions of the optic chiasm cause bitemporal hemianopias.
B. True – Macular sparing can occur if only the cortex is damaged.
C. True.
D. True – Meyer's loop: optic radiation axons that carry information from the upper part of the contralateral visual field, loop into temporal lobe en route to striate cortex.
E. True – With pituitary lesions the upper fields are affected first.

2.22

A. True – Ruffini's endings are receptive to pressure, touch and temperature. The dorsal columns transmit all three tactile sensations.
B. False – Spinothalamic pathways terminate in the intra-laminar nuclei of the thalamus.
C. True – They synapse here on second-order neurones.
D. False – It is the second-order neurones arising in the cuneate and gracile nuclei that decussate in the medial lemniscus.
E. True – Merkel's disks are receptive to pressure and touch.

2.23 Typical symptoms of normal pressure hydrocephalus include:
A. Intermittent incontinence.
B. Gait disturbance.
C. Blurred vision.
D. Occipital headaches.
E. Cognitive impairment.

2.24 The following are recognized features of dementia pugilistica (boxing encephalopathy):
A. Neurofibrillary tangles.
B. Septum pellucidum perforation.
C. Corpus callosum thinning.
D. Substantia nigra depigmentation.
E. Dysarthria.

2.25 Epileptic seizures:
A. Are followed by a drop in prolactin blood levels.
B. Are more likely following psychosurgery.
C. Contra-indicate the use of moclobemide.
D. Are in the majority of cases caused by head injury.
E. Reduce the likelihood of depression.

2.23

    A. True.
    B. True – Ataxia.
    C. False.
    D. False.
    E. True.

Note: Obstructive communicating hydrocephalus (normal-pressure hydrocephalus) is an important disorder to detect as it can be treated by shunting the dilated ventricles to the peritoneum or left atrium. The classic triad is that of incontinence, cognitive decline and ataxia. There is often no predisposing cause but in many cases there is a history of meningitis, subarachnoid haemorrhage or trauma.

2.24

    A. True – Alzheimer-like neurofibrillary tangles and plaques can be seen.
    B. True – The brain atrophies and shows contusions in proportion to the extent of exposure to blows and this occurs more so in boxers that are light-weight. Consequently there is progressive intellectual deterioration.
    C. True.
    D. True – Results in characteristic Parkinsonian slowness and rigidity.
    E. True.

2.25

    A. False – Blood prolactin levels are raised.
    B. True – The risk of seizures following psychosurgery is increased.
    C. False.
    D. False – Most cases are idiopathic. Head injury accounts for about 6–7% of cases.
    E. False – The development of depression is more likely and the risk of suicide is increased 4–5 fold.

2.26 Microglia:
- A. Have plenty of granular cytoplasm, a large rounded nucleus and flattened processes called pedicles.
- B. Are derived from haematopoetic stem cells.
- C. Form more than two-thirds of all glia.
- D. Are found predominantly in white matter.
- E. Proliferate following injury or inflammation.

2.27 The cerebral cortex:
- A. Is a derivative of the telencephalon.
- B. Is almost one-third neocortex (neopallium).
- C. Grey matter varies in thickness from 1 to 4 cm.
- D. Contains Betz cells.
- E. Is involved in the visual light reflex.

2.28 The pathology of Huntington's disease characteristically includes:
- A. Adrenal gland hypertrophy.
- B. A marked reduction of glutamic acid decarboxylase activity.
- C. Caudate nucleus atrophy.
- D. An increase in striatal aspartate receptors.
- E. An increase in neuropeptide Y levels.

2.29 EEG theta activity is diminished by the following:
- A. Alzheimer's disease.
- B. Tricyclic antidepressants.
- C. Hypoxia.
- D. Neuroleptics.
- E. Benzodiazepines.

2.26

A. False – This describes protoplasmic astrocytes. Microglia are small with elongated nuclei and have little cytoplasm.
B. True.
C. False – Form approximately 10% of all glia.
D. False – are found predominantly in grey matter.
E. True.

2.27

A. True.
B. False – 90% of the cerebral cortex is neocortex.
C. False – Varies from 1.5 to 4.5 mm.
D. True – Giant pyramidal cells found in precentral motor cortex.
E. False – Cerebral cortex is involved in accommodation reflex.

2.28

A. False – This is a finding in patients with major depression.
B. True – reduced by up to 85%.
C. True – Particularly the head of the caudate. Begins medially and eventually interrupts cortico-pallido-thalamic connections.
D. False – These are reduced.
E. True.

2.29

A. False – 95% of those with a diagnosis of Alzheimer's disease have an abnormal EEG. EEG theta and delta activity increase.
B. False – Tricyclics, benzodiazepines and neuroleptics all increase EEG theta activity.
C. False – Occipital alpha rhythm is gradually replaced by theta and delta activity. Severe hypoxia results in 'burst-suppression' effect and eventually a flat EEG.
D. False.
E. False.

2.30 The following statements are true:
A. Phospholipids are amphipathic.
B. Cerebrosides are brain proteins.
C. Water diffuses freely through biological membranes.
D. Tonic receptors continue firing as long as the stimulus lasts.
E. Free nerve endings have a low threshold of activation.

2.31 Monoamine oxidase (MAO):
A. Is found in glial mitochondria.
B. Degrades both dopamine and noradrenaline.
C. Type A (MAO-A) is not inhibited by tranylcypromine.
D. Type A (MAO-A) is found in platelets.
E. Activity in platelets is raised in schizophrenia.

2.32 Catechol-*O*-methyl-transferase (COMT):
A. Is found in the synaptic cleft.
B. Exists in both soluble and membrane-bound forms.
C. Is a manganese-dependent enzyme.
D. Is inhibited by tropolone.
E. In the brain is found predominantly in neurones.

2.30

A. True – Phospholipids and glycolipids are amphipathic. They are molecules that posses both hydrophobic and hydrophilic components.
B. False – Cerebrosides are lipids that are found mainly in myelin sheaths.
C. True – It is water-soluble molecules that have difficulty in diffusing across biological membranes.
D. True – They are slow to adapt.
E. False – It is relatively high.

2.31

A. True – MAO is found in the outer membrane of neuronal and glial mitochondria.
B. True – It degrades monoamines.
C. False – Tranylcypromine is non-specific and inhibits both MAO-A and MAO-B.
D. False – MAO-B is found in platelets. Its levels are relatively stable, although with time there is a gradual increase.
E. False – MAO activity is generally low. Indeed, low platelet MAO has been implicated in the dopamine and trans-methylation hypotheses of schizophrenia.

2.32

A. True – COMT is found in the brain, liver, kidney and heart.
B. True – In most organs it is in soluble form.
C. False – It is a Mg^{2+}-dependent enzyme.
D. True – Also by entacapone and pyrogallol.
E. False – In the brain COMT is mainly extra-neuronal and in soluble form. It is found in glial cells, ependymal cells and CSF secreting cells of the choroid plexus.

2.33 Serotonin:
A. In the body is predominantly found in blood platelets.
B. Is found in the raphe nucleus of the brainstem.
C. Is a precursor of melatonin.
D. Is metabolized by monoamine oxidase.
E. Synthesis is inhibited by *p*-chloroamphetamine (PCA).

2.34 Glutamate:
A. Is an essential amino acid.
B. Is an excitatory amino acid neurotransmitter.
C. Is converted to glutamine.
D. Is metabolized to α-ketoglutarate.
E. Is found in the hippocampus.

2.33

A. False – Serotonin (5-hydroxytryptamine) is found in many tissues of the body. Approximately 90% is found in the mucous membranes of the gastrointestinal system and about 8% in plasma platelets. Less than 2% is found in the central nervous system with small amounts in skin, lungs, liver and spleen.

B. True – It is also found in high concentration in the pineal gland.

C. True.

D. True – Undergoes oxidative deamination to form an aldehyde which is then oxidized to give 5-hydroxyindoleacetic acid (5-HIAA).

E. True – PCA, *p*-chlorophenylalanine (PCPA) and 6-fluorotryptophan all inhibit tryptophan hydroxylase, the rate-limiting enzyme in serotonin synthesis.

2.34

A. False – It can be synthesized from α-ketoglutarate by transamination or from glutamine through the action of glutaminase.

B. True – It satisfies many of the necessary criteria: localization to presynaptic vesicles, release is calcium-dependent and synaptic effects are rapidly terminated by specific re-uptake.

C. True – Glutamine synthetase converts glutamate to glutamine.

D. True – This can be achieved by either transamination or oxidative deamination.

E. True – It is thought to be important in learning and memory and in particular long-term potentiation (LTP).

2.35 During pregnancy the risk of increased frequency of seizures can be reliably predicted from:
A. The duration of epilepsy.
B. The type of seizures.
C. Family history.
D. The relationship of seizures to the menstrual cycle.
E. The frequency of seizures in previous pregnancies.

2.36 Thioridazine:
A. Causes orthostatic hypotension through α_1 adrenoceptor blockade.
B. Interacts with post-synaptic mesolimbic and mesocortical D2 receptors.
C. When prescribed at high doses for long periods of time can cause pigmentary retinopathy.
D. Is a piperidine side-chain thioxanthene.
E. Can be administered by deep intramuscular injection.

2.37 The following drugs are tertiary amine tricyclic antidepressants (TCAs):
A. Nortriptyline.
B. Maprotiline.
C. Doxepin.
D. Mianserin.
E. Trimipramine.

2.35

    A. False.
    B. False.
    C. False.
    D. False.
    E. False.

Note: Seizure frequency is increased in approximately 5–50% of cases and it is most likely to occur in the first two trimesters of pregnancy. This increase is usually related to sleep deprivation or changes in plasma drug levels of anti-epileptic medication. The only observation of any predictive value is that women with poorly controlled epilepsy prior to pregnancy are more likely to suffer poor control during pregnancy.

2.36

    A. True – α_1 adrenoceptor blockade causes orthostatic hypotension and ejaculatory failure.
    B. True – This is thought to be responsible for its clinical antipsychotic effect.
    C. True – With prolonged use, regular eye examinations are necessary.
    D. False – It is a piperidine side-chain phenothiazine.
    E. False – Available only as oral preparations (tablets and syrup).

2.37

    A. False.
    B. False.
    C. True.
    D. False.
    E. True.

Note: Tricyclics have a three-ring nucleus and a side-chain. The number of methyl groups attached to the nitrogen atom of the side-chain determine whether a TCA is described as secondary (one group) or tertiary (two groups) amines.

Tertiary amine TCAs are amitriptyline, imipramine, trimipramine, clomipramine and doxepin. Secondary amine TCAs are nortriptyline, desipramine, protriptyline.

Mianserin and maprotiline are tetracyclic drugs.

2.38 The following statements concerning SSRIs are true:
A. Citalopram is indicated for use in panic disorder.
B. Norfluoxetine is an active metabolite of fluoxetine.
C. Fluvoxamine is not metabolized and undergoes renal elimination unchanged.
D. Paroxetine does not lower the seizure threshold.
E. Sertraline is tightly bound to plasma proteins.

2.39 The following statements about congenital abnormalities are correct:
A. 50% of foetuses have chromosomal abnormalities and the majority of these abort.
B. One in 400 pregnancies results in the birth of a child with a congenital abnormality.
C. The cause of most congenital abnormalities is unknown.
D. 0.5% of live new-born infants have chromosomal abnormalities.
E. The risk of a Down's syndrome infant being born to a 20-year-old mother is 1 in 20 000.

2.40 In DNA replication:
A. Synthesis can only take place $3' \rightarrow 5'$
B. DNA polymerase δ conducts synthesis along the leading strand.
C. Okazaki fragments are used along the lagging strand.
D. The process (complete DNA replication) is complete within 8 minutes.
E. The process is described as semi-discontinuous.

2.41 Stigmata of Down's syndrome include:
A. Endocardial cushion defects.
B. Brachycephalic skull.
C. Clinodactyly.
D. Cataracts.
E. Fissured tongue.

2.38

  A. True – Citalopram and paroxetine are both indicated for use in panic disorder.
  B. True – Fluoxetine is metabolized to norfluoxetine in the liver. Whereas fluoxetine has a half-life of 2–3 days, norfluoxetine has a half-life of 1 week and is eventually eliminated by the kidneys.
  C. False – All the SSRIs are readily metabolized.
  D. True – It also has little effect on psychomotor skills but does cause nausea, headaches and somnolescence. Clinically it is also noted to have a marked withdrawal syndrome.
  E. True.

2.39

  A. False – Only 5% of foetuses have chromosomal abnormalities.
  B. False – One in 40 pregnancies results in the birth of a child with a congenital abnormality.
  C. True – The aetiology can be genetic, environmental or multifactorial.
  D. True – Autosomal chromosomes are twice as likely to be affected as sex chromosomes.
  E. False – 1 in 2000.

2.40

  A. False – Only in opposite direction, i.e. $5' \rightarrow 3'$.
  B. True – DNA polymerase α acts along lagging strand.
  C. True – These are then joined together by DNA ligase.
  D. False – Approximately 8 hours.
  E. True – And also semi-conservative.

2.41

  A. True – Occur in 40–50%.
  B. True – With flat occiput.
  C. True – Occurs in 50%. Also have abnormal dermatoglyphics.
  D. True.
  E. True – Tongue is also unusually large.

2.42 Recognized features of Turner's syndrome include:
A. Prognathia.
B. Receding hairline.
C. Coarctation of the aorta.
D. Cubitus varus.
E. Lymphoedema.

2.43 Opioid receptors:
A. Include μ (mu), δ (delta) and κ (kappa) receptors.
B. Are metabotropic.
C. Activate adenylate cyclase.
D. Are antagonized by naloxone.
E. Are involved in analgesia.

2.44 Somatostatin:
A. Facilitates the release of glucagon from the pancreas.
B. Inhibits the release of thyroid-stimulating hormone.
C. Cortical concentration is diminished in Alzheimer's disease.
D. Peaks in slow-wave sleep.
E. Corpus striatum concentration is diminished in Huntington's disease.

2.42

A. False – Cranio-facial abnormalities include micrognathia, low-set ears, webbed neck and downward slanting palpebral fissures.
B. False – A recognized feature is a low hairline at the back of the head.
C. True – Other cardiovascular defects include atrial septal defects and hypertension.
D. False – It is cubitus valgus (wide carrying angle).
E. True.

2.43

A. True – These are the three main groups of receptors. Others that are described include ϵ (epsilon) receptors and σ (sigma) receptors. However, the latter are probably not opiate receptors as they are not blocked by traditional opiate antagonists and are thought to be associated with the NMDA receptor.
B. True – They are G-protein coupled and inhibit neurotransmission.
C. False – They inhibit adenylate cyclase.
D. True – And also by naltrexone. These can be used in the treatment of opiate addiction.
E. True – Opiate receptors and opioids are thought to be important in thermoregulation, movement disorders, learning and memory and addiction.

2.44

A. False – Somatostatin suppresses the release of glucagon and insulin in the pancreas.
B. True – It also inhibits the release of growth hormone.
C. True.
D. True – Thought to be important in both slow-wave and REM sleep.
E. False – Levels are increased.

2.45 Cholecystokinin:
- A. Stimulates appetite.
- B. Coexists with dopamine in the nucleus accumbens.
- C. Is a glycoprotein.
- D. Is present in the hippocampus.
- E. Inhibits the secretion of pancreatic enzymes.

2.46 Measures of dispersion:
- A. The range can be applied to nominal values.
- B. The variance uses all the values in the distribution.
- C. The units used to express standard deviation are the square of those of the data.
- D. The standard error of the mean measures the extent of variation of the sample means.
- E. The coefficient of variation is an absolute measure of dispersion.

2.47 Correlation:
- A. Pearson's product – moment correlation coefficient has the same units as the data.
- B. Spearman's rank correlation coefficient can only be applied to normally distributed variables.
- C. Examines the extent to which two variables are causally related.
- D. Can be assessed using regression analysis.
- E. Is usually expressed along a scale 0 to 1.

2.48 Magnetic resonance imaging (MRI):
- A. Has a slice resolution of < 1 mm.
- B. Measures proton density.
- C. Is contra-indicated in pregnancy.
- D. Is better at discriminating grey and white matter than computerized tomography.
- E. Precession refers to the return of nuclei to their previous quantum level resulting in the emission of radio frequency waves.

2.45

A. False – It is associated with satiety.
B. True – It is also colocalized with dopamine in the ventral tegmental area of the brain stem.
C. False – It is a gut – brain polypeptide. CCK-8 is the most prevalent form.
D. True – Also found in the amygdala and cerebral cortex.
E. False – It stimulates the secretion of pancreatic enzymes and increases gall-bladder motility.

2.46

A. False – It can only be applied to values measured on an interval or ratio scale.
B. True – It calculates their deviation from the mean.
C. False – This is true for variance. The units of standard deviation are the same as those of the data.
D. True – It is calculated by dividing the standard deviation by the square root of the sample size.
E. True – It is not expressed in any units and therefore allows comparison of dispersions.

2.47

A. False – It has no units.
B. False.
C. False – Causality is not implied by correlation.
D. True.
E. False – Usually expressed along a scale of -1 to $+1$.

2.48

A. True.
B. True.
C. True.
D. True.
E. False – This is termed relaxation. Precession refers to the axial rotation that is specific to each atom.

2.49 Functional neuroimaging:

A. Positron emission tomography (PET) relies on the use of ligands labelled radioactively with a gamma photon emitting isotope.

B. Functional magnetic resonance imaging relies on blood oxygenation level to map cortical activation.

C. Single photon emission computed tomography (SPECT) requires the use of an on-site cyclotron.

D. Magnetic encephalography is useful for localizing epileptiform activity.

E. Includes magnetic resonance spectroscopy.

2.50 Positron emission tomography (PET):

A. Has a resolution of 1–2 mm.

B. Most commonly uses isotopes ^{18}F, ^{15}O and ^{13}N.

C. The half-life of the isotopes used is 24–72 hours.

D. Is immune to Compton scattering.

E. Resolution is affected by signal attenuation.

2.49

    A.   False – This is the basis of SPECT.

    B.   True – Sometimes called the BOLD (Blood Oxygen Level Dependent) effect.

    C.   False – A cyclotron is necessary for PET in order to create positrons.

    D.   True.

    E.   True.

2.50

    A.   False – Much less, i.e. 5–6 mm.

    B.   True – Particularly fluorine-18-deoxyglucose.

    C.   False – A matter of minutes to a couple of hours only.

    D.   False.

    E.   True.

Paper 3

3.1 Instrumental learning:
A. Is based on Thorndike's Law of Effect.
B. Involves respondent behaviour.
C. Was used by Watson and Rayner to induce a white rat phobia in Little Albert.
D. Involves operant behaviour.
E. Is studied using maze-learning paradigms.

3.2 Gestalt principles of perception include:
A. Prolixity.
B. Continuity.
C. Complexity.
D. Reversibility.
E. Conservation.

3.3 Long-term memory:
A. Is also described as tertiary memory.
B. Has finite capacity.
C. Coding is solely acoustic.
D. Storage and retrieval require more effort than short-term memory.
E. Is described as declarative and procedural.

3.4 The following statements are true:
A. The interference of prior learning with subsequent learning is called proactive inhibition.
B. In Hull's drive-reduction theory of motivation anxiety is considered a primary drive.
C. Drives are physiological and can be defined objectively.
D. The need for achievement is a behavioural model of motivation described by McClelland.
E. In Maslow's hierarchy of needs aesthetic needs must be satisfied before cognitive needs can be addressed.

3.1

   A. True – Behaviour is controlled by its consequences, and behaviour that is successful is rewarded and strengthened and therefore more likely to be repeated.

   B. True – Behaviour that is caused directly by environmental events.

   C. False – They utilized classical conditioning.

   D. True.

   E. True – For example, radial arm maze and Morris water maze.

3.2

   A. False – Prolixity refers to a flight of ideas in which a train of thought eventually returns to its original track.

   B. True.

   C. False – Converse is true. Simplicity.

   D. False.

   E. False.

Note: Correct responses include similarity, closure, simplicity, continuity and proximity.

3.3

   A. False – Also described as secondary memory.

   B. False – Theoretically unlimited capacity. Limited by retrieval.

   C. False – Can also be visual or semantic.

   D. True.

   E. True – Declarative (knowing that) and procedural (knowing how).

3.4

   A. True – As opposed to retroactive inhibition.

   B. False – It is secondary (acquired) drive. Primary drives are innate, e.g. hunger.

   C. False – They are psychological, hypothetical constructs. Needs are physiological and produce drives.

   D. False – It is a cognitive model of motivation.

   E. False – The reverse is true. The order from more basic to more sophisticated needs is: physiological, safety, social, esteem, cognitive, aesthetic and finally self-actualization.

3.5 The following statements are true:
  A. Complex messages are persuasive in intelligent recipients with high self-esteem.
  B. Heider's balance theory states that when two attitudes are mutually inconsistent the one that is less firmly held will change.
  C. Implicit messages are more persuasive for intelligent recipients.
  D. One-sided uncritical presentation is best suited to an intelligent audience.
  E. Fearful message is better at influencing those with high levels of anxiety.

3.6 Interpersonal attraction is increased by:
  A. Novelty.
  B. Separation.
  C. Familiarity.
  D. Reciprocal self-disclosure.
  E. Perceived competence.

3.7 The following statements are correct:
  A. The matching hypothesis states that opposites attract.
  B. Schizophrenic individuals have larger personal space.
  C. Exchange theory proposes that individuals most prefer relationships that are costly but have high rewards.
  D. Equity theory proposes that relationships are viewed as property.
  E. The fundamental attribution error involves individuals attributing the behaviour of others to situational causes.

3.8 Social influence:
  A. Task performance is enhanced by the presence of others.
  B. Task performance is diminished by the presence of others.
  C. The effect of others on task performance is known as bystander intervention.
  D. According to social impact theory the degree of social influence in a particular situation is a function of the total number of people exerting the influence.
  E. In situations of urgency the diffusion of responsibility is helpful to the individual in need.

3.5
A. True.
B. False – This is Osgood and Tannenbaum's congruity theory. Heider's balance theory proposes that individuals seek harmony of attitudes and beliefs and evaluate related things in a similar manner.
C. True.
D. False – Two-sided presentation is better suited to an informed, intelligent audience.
E. False – This is better at influencing recipients with low levels of anxiety.

3.6
A. False – Increased by similarity.
B. False – Increased by proximity.
C. True.
D. True.
E. True.
Note: Also important are physical attractiveness and reciprocal liking.

3.7
A. False – The matching hypothesis suggests that individuals pair with those of equivalent attractiveness and are matched in terms of mutual reward.
B. True – As do violent criminals.
C. False – Preference is for relationships that offer the greatest gains with least expense.
D. False – This introduces the concept of fairness with approximately equal gains in the relationship for both individuals.
E. False – Personal behaviour is attributed to situational factors whereas that of others is attributed to internal causes.

3.8
A. True – But can also be diminished.
B. True – Complex or novel tasks or hostility from others can adversely affect performance.
C. False – It is called the 'audience effect'.
D. True – It is also dependent upon strength and immediacy.
E. False – This and pluralistic ignorance serve to promote inaction and are therefore unhelpful.

3.9 The following statements concerning reliability and testing are correct:
- A. Split-half reliability: signifies the stability of a test or measure.
- B. Inter-rater reliability: the degree of agreement between different raters assessing the same parameters within the same time-frame.
- C. Test–retest reliability: signifies the internal consistency of a measure or test.
- D. Sensitivity: the degree to which a test or measure is able to distinguish and exclude those without the property that it determines.
- E. Positive predictive value: the proportion correctly described by a test as positive.

3.10 Definitions of intelligence:
- A. Sternberg described fluid ability and crystallized ability.
- B. Hebb described genetically based potential and effective intelligence.
- C. Spearman described component intelligence and experiential intelligence.
- D. Thurstone proposed primary mental abilities.
- E. Cattell developed the concept of general intelligence factor (g).

3.11 In the spectrum of normal temperamental patterns, *difficult children*:
- A. Form the largest group.
- B. Are regular in habits.
- C. Are slow to adapt.
- D. Show emotional lability.
- E. Find it difficult to cry.

3.12 In Piaget's model of cognitive development:
- A. New experiences outside of existing schemata produce disequilibrium.
- B. New schemas are developed by assimilation.
- C. Accommodation refers to the adjustment of existing schemas to facilitate comprehension of new information.
- D. The process of understanding through assimilation and accommodation is termed triangulation.
- E. Children think differently to adults.

3.9

A. False – This applies to test–retest reliability.
B. True.
C. False – This applies to split-half reliability.
D. False – This is the specificity. Sensitivity is the degree to which a test is able to detect the property that it determines.
E. True.

3.10

A. False – Cattell.
B. True – Type A and Type B.
C. False – Sternberg.
D. True – Memory, number, word fluency, perceptual speed, verbal comprehension, reasoning and space.
E. False – Spearman.

3.11

A. False – They only make up 10% of all children, easy children make up 40%.
B. False – This is a feature of easy children.
C. True – This is also true of those children described as slow-to-warm-up.
D. True – They are also difficult to comfort.
E. False – They react intensely and cry easily.

3.12

A. True.
B. False – Assimilation refers to incorporation of new/ novel information into existing schemas.
C. True.
D. False – It is termed circular reaction.
E. True – For instance, children display egocentrism: they are unable to distinguish their personal perspective.

3.13 Psychiatric patients from poor socio-economic background are more likely to be:
A. Admitted to hospital.
B. Schizophrenic.
C. Treated with ECT.
D. Alcohol dependent.
E. Suffering from eating disorders.

3.14 Dream work, according to Freud, involves the following:
A. Reversal.
B. Secondary elaboration.
C. Displacement.
D. Condensation.
E. Symbolization.

3.15 The following are Jungian archetypes:
A. Libido.
B. Shadow.
C. Complex.
D. Self.
E. Personal unconscious.

3.13

    A.   True – And remain in-patients for longer.

    B.   True.

    C.   True – And pharmacotherapy.

    D.   True.

    E.   False – Psychiatric disorders more commonly diagnosed in the higher social classes are bipolar disorder and eating disorders.

3.14

    A.   False – The latent dream is transformed into the manifest dream through mechanisms of dream work. Reversal is a defence mechanism in which an instinct though maintaining its aim is reversed in its choice of object.

    B.   True – The revision/rationalization that occurs upon waking.

    C.   True – The latent content is replaced by obscurely related elements.

    D.   True – Latent elements are fused.

    E.   True – The use of symbols to represent abstract ideas.

3.15

    A.   False – In Jungian theory the libido stems from all psychic energy and life. Archetypes are contents of the collective unconscious which are manifest as archetypal images and have symbolic meaning.

    B.   True – This is the unconscious counterpart of the ego and consists of repressed primitive animal instincts.

    C.   False – Complexes surround archetypes and are networks of ideas and thoughts that are linked through commonality of emotions and feelings.

    D.   True – Binds conscious and unconscious elements and is the goal of individuation. It develops as the individual deals with other archetypes.

    E.   False – This is relatively superficial. It is the objective psyche (collective conscious) that gives rise to consciousness.

3.16 Donald Winnicott:
   A. Formulated the concept of a *transitional space*.
   B. Founded the humanistic school of psychology.
   C. Trained initially as a paediatrician.
   D. Described the *good-enough mother*.
   E. Used the term *psychological games* to describe the interaction between mother and child.

3.17 The following definitions are correct:
   A. Overvalued idea: a fixed false belief that is not in keeping with the individual's cultural background or the beliefs of their peers.
   B. Nihilistic delusion: delusional belief of negation.
   C. Apophanous perception: novel delusional interpretation of a normal perception which cannot be completely understood in terms of the patient's mental state.
   D. Syndrome of Fregoli: familiar person is falsely identified in complete strangers.
   E. Eidetic image: spontaneous, false perception occurring in objective space with the full force of a real perception in the absence of a real stimulus or object.

3.18 The following definitions are correct:
   A. Capgras syndrome: individual believes that a closely related or familiar person has been supplanted by an imposter who is an exact double.
   B. Pareidolia: visual hallucination that occurs in dim light.
   C. Gedankenlautwerden: running commentary auditory hallucination.
   D. Elementary hallucination: pseudohallucination.
   E. Extracampine hallucination: perceived outside of individual's field of perception.

3.19 Cranial nerves:
   A. The facial nerve supplies the muscles of the first pharyngeal arch.
   B. Impulses from the utricle are transmitted towards the brain in the vestibular nerve.
   C. In conduction deafness the sound of a vibrating tuning fork placed at the vertex is louder in the normal ear.
   D. The sensory arc of the gag reflex involves the glosso-pharyngeal nerve.
   E. The spinal accessory nerve supplies the soft palate.

3.16

A. True – It is in this space that the transitional object functions.
B. False – Gordon Allport founded the humanistic school of psychology.
C. True.
D. True – This is a mother that is responsive to the baby's needs and manages to balance gratification and frustration.
E. False – This term was used by Eric Berne to describe the interaction between the various ego states of an individual (child, adult, parent).

3.17

A. False – This describes a delusion.
B. True.
C. True – Delusional perception.
D. True – Reciprocal of Capgras.
E. False – This describes a hallucination. Eidetic image is the recollection of a memory as a hallucination, reproducing a vivid perception.

3.18

A. True.
B. False – It is a vivid, effortless illusion.
C. False – Auditory hallucination involving own thoughts spoken aloud.
D. False – Basic sounds, noises and whistles. Nevertheless true hallucinations.
E. True.

3.19

A. False – It is the nerve of the second pharyngeal arch.
B. True – The utricle, saccule and semicircular canals are involved in maintaining balance.
C. False – Weber test; with conduction deafness the sound is louder in the affected ear.
D. True.
E. True – Cranial root also supplies the larynx and pharynx.

3.20 The following are associated with optic neuritis:
A. Sarcoidosis.
B. Syphilis.
C. Gonorrhoea.
D. Oral contraceptives.
E. Multiple sclerosis.

3.21 Causes of Wernicke–Korsakov syndrome include:
A. Thiamine deficiency.
B. Carbon monoxide poisoning.
C. Gastric carcinoma.
D. Ventricular tumours.
E. Mamillary body damage.

3.22 Alzheimer's disease neuritic plaques:
A. Contain β-amyloid derived from amyloid precursor protein.
B. Are intracellular.
C. Are present in normal ageing brains.
D. Correlate more closely than neurofibrillary tangles with disease severity.
E. Consist of paired helical filaments.

3.23 Recognized clinical and pathological findings in patients with schizophrenia include:
A. The increase in ventricular size is more marked in males.
B. The amygdala is reduced in size.
C. There is a greater incidence of cavum septum pellucidum.
D. Prefrontal cortex neuronal density is reduced.
E. Both pursuit and saccadic eye movements are abnormal.

3.20

  A. True.
  B. True.
  C. False.
  D. False.
  E. True – The retrobulbar portion of the optic nerve (long segment behind the eye) is susceptible to inflammation. This is called retrobulbar or optic neuritis. It is painful and can lead to loss of vision. It is particularly common in multiple sclerosis and is also caused by vasculitis, tobacco and ethyl and methyl alcohol.

3.21

  A. True – This is usually because of alcohol abuse. Hyperemsis and gastric carcinoma also lead to thiamine deficiency.
  B. True.
  C. True.
  D. True – Tumours of the fourth ventricle.
  E. True – Petechial haemorrhages, parenchymal degeneration and capillary proliferation within grey matter surrounding third and fourth ventricles.

3.22

  A. True – The amyloid precursor protein gene is located on the long arm of chromosome 21.
  B. False – They are extracellular.
  C. True – Also in CJD and Down's syndrome.
  D. False – The reverse is true.
  E. False – These are found in neurofibrillary tangles not plaques.

3.23

  A. True – Lateral and third ventricles are enlarged.
  B. True – The hippocampus is also reduced in size (changes more marked on left).
  C. True – The septum pellucidum is increased in size.
  D. True – Neuronal density is also diminished in anterior cingulate and primary motor cortices and mediodorsal thalamic nucleus and nucleus accumbens.
  E. True.

3.24 The following are associated with excessive salivation or drooling:
A. Sjögren's syndrome.
B. Parkinson's disease.
C. Anxiety.
D. Clozapine.
E. Wilson's disease.

3.25 Temporal lobe:
A. Atrophy occurs in Pick's disease.
B. Grey matter volume is diminished in schizophrenia.
C. Functions include olfactory processing.
D. Insular cortex contains the gyri of Heschl.
E. Lesions usually result in bitemporal hemianopia.

3.26 Argyll–Robertson pupils:
A. React to light.
B. Are of irregular shape.
C. Are characteristically associated with ptosis.
D. Are asymmetric.
E. Are unresponsive to accommodation.

3.24

A. False – Sjögren's syndrome is a recognized cause of xerostomia and it is characterized by dryness of eyes, mouth and skin.
B. True – Often leads to drooling.
C. False – Usually causes dryness of the mouth.
D. True – Recognized and troublesome side-effect.
E. True.

3.25

A. True – Pick's disease causes marked asymmetrical fronto-temporal atrophy with notable sparing of the posterior one-third of the superior temporal gyrus.
B. True – Medial temporal structures, e.g. parahippocampal gyrus and hippocampus have been shown to be reduced in volume (change is more marked on left side of brain).
C. True – The uncus and adjoining parts of the parahippocampal gyrus contain the olfactory receptive area. Damage to this area can result in anosmia and irritative foci can cause uncinate fits.
D. True – The anterior transverse temporal gyri of Heschl lie within the embedded portion of the superior temporal cortex called the insula.
E. False – Bitemporal hemianopia is usually indicative of optic chiasma pathology. Deep temporal lobe lesions interrupt the optic radiation resulting in contralateral homonymous upper quadrantic visual field defects.

3.26

A. False – They are characteristically unresponsive to light.
B. True – They are small, asymmetrical and irregular.
C. False – Found in oculomotor nerve palsy and Horner's syndrome.
D. True – Caused by diabetic autonomic neuropathy and syphilis.
E. False.

3.27 Telencephalon derivatives include:
A. Pons.
B. Cerebral aqueduct of Sylvius.
C. Hippocampus.
D. Thalamus.
E. Basal ganglia.

3.28 Huntington's disease:
A. Affects 1 in 2000 people.
B. Is caused by a deletion on chromosome 4.
C. Produces 'bat-wing' ventricles.
D. Causes cortical neuronal loss from layers 3, 5 and 6.
E. Is associated with a loss of striatal substance P.

3.29 Primary cerebral tumours:
A. Are less common than metastases (secondary cerebral tumours).
B. Are most commonly ectodermal in origin.
C. In adults are mainly infratentorial.
D. Are usually multiple.
E. Have a characteristically diffuse growing edge.

3.30 Bombesin:
A. Is functionally related to kinesin.
B. Is found in the hypothalamus.
C. Lowers blood pressure.
D. Is a potent appetite stimulant.
E. Stimulates the release of prolactin and growth hormone.

3.27

A. False – The pons is a derivative of the metencephalon.
B. False – This is derived from the mesencephalon.
C. True – Derivatives of the telencephalon (forebrain) include the cerebral hemispheres, hippocampus, basal ganglia, olfactory bulb and lateral ventricles.
D. False – The thalamus, subthalamus, epithalamus and hypothalamus are all parts of the diencephalon.
E. True.

3.28

A. False – It affects 1 in 20 000 people, men and women equally.
B. False – It is an autosomal dominant genetic disorder caused by excessive trinucleotide (CAG) repeats on short arm of chromosome 4.
C. True – The ventricles are enlarged and can produce this pattern.
D. True – Neuronal degeneration and loss is associated with marked astrocytosis.
E. True – Substance P containing neurones project to the substantia nigra.

3.29

A. False – 80% of cerebral tumours are primary and only 20% are secondary.
B. False – The majority are neuroepithelial and mesodermal in origin.
C. False – In adults 70% are supratentorial and the reverse is true in infants and children.
D. False – It is metastases that are usually multiple.
E. True.

3.30

A. False – Kinesin is an ATPase that is structurally similar to myosin. It is involved in axonal transport.
B. True – It is found in high concentrations in hypothalamus, midbrain and cortex.
C. False – It raises blood pressure and is involved in thermoregulation.
D. False – It inhibits feeding.
E. True – It is also antidiuretic.

3.31 In chemical synaptic neurotransmission:
  A. Arrival at the synaptic bouton of the presynaptic action potential results in calcium efflux.
  B. A conjoint synapse is one which also has electrical characteristics.
  C. Neurotransmitter vesicles are released at specific presynaptic sites called gap junctions.
  D. There is a synaptic delay.
  E. Synapses are unidirectional.

3.32 Gamma-aminobutyric acid (GABA):
  A. Concentration in caudate neurones is increased in Huntington's disease.
  B. Metabolism by GABA aminotransferase is inhibited by vigabatrin.
  C. Is synthesized from glutamate.
  D. Is highly concentrated in peripheral nervous system sympathetic ganglia.
  E. Readily crosses the blood–brain barrier.

3.33 Glycine:
  A. Contains an α-carbon atom.
  B. Is not found in spinal cord tissue.
  C. Is synthesized in a single reaction from serine.
  D. Is described as an excitatory amino acid neurotransmitter.
  E. Is a catecholamine.

3.31

A. False – Calcium influx takes place and this initiates presynaptic vesicle migration and fusion.
B. True.
C. False – Gap junctions are electrical synapses. In these there is direct membranous contact and neurotransmission is faster.
D. True – This is usually about 1 ms.
E. True.

3.32

A. False – The concentration of GABA in caudate neurones is < 50% of normal in those with Huntington's disease. This is accompanied by a marked reduction of glutamic acid decarboxylase activity.
B. True.
C. True – GABA is synthesized in a single reaction from glutamate. The reaction is catalysed by glutamate (glutamic acid) decarboxylase.
D. False – GABA is found only in trace amounts in many peripheral tissues (liver, spleen and heart) and nerves including sympathetic ganglia. Within the CNS its concentration is in the order of μmoles/g rather than nmoles/g as in the case of monoamines.
E. False.

3.33

A. False – It is the only amino acid not to possess an α-carbon atom (a carbon atom to which there are four different chemical groups attached).
B. False – It is found in spinal cord tissue particularly Renshaw cells which inhibit motor neurones via the inhibitory actions of glycine.
C. True – This is catalysed by serine hydroxymethyltransferase.
D. False – It is, along with GABA, an inhibitory amino acid neurotransmitter.
E. False – Glycine has a very simple chemical structure with two hydrogen atoms attached to the amine-carboxyl group backbone ($NH_3^+CH_2COO^-$).

3.34 D$_2$ receptors:
A. Are present in the caudate nucleus.
B. Are functionally grouped with D$_5$ receptors.
C. Bind bromocriptine.
D. Are ionotropic receptors.
E. Possess both pre- and post-synaptic functions.

3.35 The following drugs are likely to cause infant toxicity by virtue of being secreted in breast milk:
A. Paracetamol.
B. Bromocriptine.
C. Ethosuximide.
D. Insulin.
E. Iodine.

3.34

A. True – Abundant in caudate and putamen, also found in nucleus accumbens, olfactory tubercles, hypothalamus and pituitary.

B. False – Dopamine receptors are broadly described as D_1-like (D_5) and D_2-like (D_3 and D_4). All are metabotropic receptors and are linked to adenylate cyclase via Gs (D_1- like) and Gi (D_2-like).

C. True – Bromocriptine is an agonist.

D. False – They are metabotropic receptors coupled to G-proteins.

E. True – D_2-like receptors have both pre- and post-synaptic actions. D_1-like receptors have only post-synaptic functions.

3.35

A. False – Amount secreted in breast milk is too small to cause any harm.

B. False – Bromocriptine is a dopamine agonist that inhibits pituitary release of prolactin. It suppresses lactation and is used for the treatment of galactorrhoea.

C. True – A significant amount is secreted in the milk. It can cause hyperexcitability in the infant and should be avoided in breast-feeding.

D. False – Amount secreted in breast milk is too small to cause any harm.

E. True – Iodine seems to be concentrated in breast milk and can cause a goitre or neonatal hypothyroidism.

Note: Infant toxicity can occur if significant amounts of a drug enter breast milk. For most drugs there is insufficient evidence in this area. Therefore, as a general rule, all but essential pharmacotherapy should be avoided in breast-feeding.

3.36 Moclobemide:
A. Can be used in the treatment of social phobia.
B. Inhibits the predominant form of monoamine oxidase in the noradrenergic neurones of the locus coeruleus.
C. Commonly causes raised liver enzymes.
D. Can be used in the treatment of phaeochromacytoma.
E. Does not necessitate a treatment-free period when switching to another antidepressant.

3.37 Lithium:
A. Is excreted in sweat.
B. Is not bound to plasma proteins.
C. Use in pregnancy is associated with Ebstein's anomaly.
D. Plasma levels are decreased by thiazide diuretics.
E. Causes hyperkalaemia.

3.38 The following statements concerning benzodiazepines are true:
A. Slow intravenous lorazepam is paradoxically helpful in acute pulmonary insufficiency.
B. Temazepam and alprazolam belong to different classes of benzodiazepines.
C. Diazepam is absorbed from the gastrointestinal tract as desmethyldiazepam.
D. Midazolam is only available in injectable form.
E. Zopiclone is a 2-keto-benzodiazepine.

Paper 3

3.36
- **A.** True.
- **B.** True – It is a reversible inhibitor of monoamine oxidase-A (MAO-A) which is the predominant form of the enzyme in the noradrenergic neurones of the locus coeruleus. The preferred substrates of MAO-A are, noradrenaline, adrenaline and dopamine.
- **C.** False – This is a rare side-effect.
- **D.** False – It is contra-indicated in phaeochromacytoma and acute confusional states.
- **E.** True – This is not necessary because of its short duration of action. However, when switching **to** moclobemide **from** other antidepressants a drug-free period is necessary: a week following most tricyclic antidepressants, 2 weeks after sertraline or paroxetine and 5 weeks or more when switching from fluoxetine.

3.37
- **A.** True – Lithium is mainly eliminated by the kidneys but it is also excreted in faeces, sweat and in breast milk.
- **B.** True.
- **C.** True – Lithium should not be prescribed in the first trimester of pregnancy because it increases the incidence of defects at birth. Ebstein's anomaly (congenital cardiac anomaly of the tricuspid valve) occurs in 3–10% of babies exposed to lithium.
- **D.** False – Distal tubule diuretics such as the thiazides increase plasma lithium levels.
- **E.** False – Usually causes hypokalaemia which may produce electrocardiogram (ECG) T-wave flattening.

3.38
- **A.** False – Benzodiazepines are contra-indicated.
- **B.** True – Temazepam is a 3-hydroxy-benzodiazepine, alprazolam is a triazolo-benzodiazepine.
- **C.** False – All the benzodiazepines are absorbed completely unchanged from the gastrointestinal tract except clorazepate which is absorbed as desmethyldiazepam.
- **D.** True – It is used mainly for premedication in anaesthetics.
- **E.** False – It is a cyclopyrrolone.

3.39 Sodium valproate:
  A. Is used in the treatment of all forms of epilepsy.
  B. Plasma levels are a useful indication of efficacy.
  C. Prescribed in the first trimester of pregnancy increases the risk of neural tube defects.
  D. Gastrointestinal absorption is reduced by the presence of food.
  E. Has a rare side-effect of pancreatitis.

3.40 Down's syndrome is associated with the following:
  A. Hyperthyroidism.
  B. Rigidity.
  C. Hirschsprung's disease.
  D. Duodenal atresia.
  E. Leukaemia.

3.41 In Turner's syndrome:
  A. 1 in 20 000 females are affected.
  B. Intelligence is largely unaffected.
  C. Diagnosis can be made by buccal mucosal cell chromosomal analysis.
  D. 50% of XO foetuses miscarry.
  E. Infertility is common.

3.42 Neurofibromatosis type 1:
  A. Is characterized by Lisch nodules.
  B. Is also called von Recklinghausen's disease.
  C. Is inherited in an autosomal dominant pattern on chromosome 22.
  D. Is characterized by bilateral acoustic neuromas.
  E. Is often the result of a new mutation.

3.39

A. True – It is also used as a second-line therapy for bipolar affective disorder.
B. False – Plasma level monitoring is occasionally useful for the detection of toxicity or the assessment of compliance. It can also be of help when more than one drug is being administered, however, routine monitoring is largely unhelpful.
C. True – Patients should be offered counselling.
D. False – The presence of food may delay absorption but it does not affect the total amount absorbed.
E. True – It can cause pancreatic failure and liver toxicity.

3.40

A. False – Hypothyroidism.
B. False – Hypotonia.
C. True.
D. True.
E. True – 1%.

3.41

A. False – 1 in 2500 female births have Turner's syndrome.
B. True – Verbal IQ is normal but performance IQ is about 90 after adolescence.
C. True.
D. False – 99% of XO foetuses miscarry.
E. True – Ovarian dysgenesis (streak ovaries) results in infertility.

3.42

A. True – These are melanocytic hamartomas that appear as multiple yellow–brown nodules on the iris.
B. True – This is the 'peripheral' type of neurofibromatosis.
C. False – It is inherited on chromosome 17.
D. False – Type 2 neurofibromatosis is characterized by bilateral acoustic neuromas. It is the 'central' type and is inherited in an autosomal dominant pattern on chromosome 22.
E. True – In almost 50% of cases it arises sporadically.

3.43 Phenylketonuria:
A. Is the most common known cause of mental retardation.
B. Arises because of an inability to absorb phenylalanine.
C. Is tested for in the first 36 hours of life using the Guthrie test.
D. Is inherited as an X-linked recessive disorder.
E. Was described by Kanner.

3.44 Vasoactive intestinal peptide (VIP):
A. Inhibits the release of prolactin.
B. Stimulates the release of growth hormone.
C. Inhibits the release of somatostatin.
D. Coexists with acetylcholine in cortical neurones.
E. Inhibits the release of ACTH.

3.45 Corticotrophin-releasing hormone (CRH):
A. Is released from the supraoptic nucleus of the hypothalamus.
B. Release is stimulated by noradrenaline.
C. Stimulates the cleavage of pro-opiomelanocortin.
D. Is a pentapeptide.
E. Binding sites are increased in the frontal cortex of suicides.

3.43

A. False – It is the third most common known cause of mental retardation (after Down's syndrome and fragile X).

B. False – It arises because of an absence of phenylalanine hydroxylase.

C. False – The levels of phenylalanine are normal at birth and the Guthrie test (uses *Bacillus subtilis* which is dependent on phenylalanine for multiplication) is best carried out in the second week of life (days 6–14).

D. False – It is inherited as an autosomal recessive disorder.

E. False – Leo Kanner described autistic disorder. Phenylketonuria was described by Folling.

3.44

A. False – It stimulates the release of prolactin, growth hormone and ACTH. Dopamine inhibits the release of prolactin.

B. True – Its actions are largely excitatory.

C. True.

D. True – VIP is found in autonomic ganglia, intestinal and respiratory tracts and in the cerebral cortex, hypothalamus, amygdala and hippocampus.

E. False.

3.45

A. False – It is released from the paraventricular nucleus of the hypothalamus.

B. True – This seems to be a reciprocal relationship.

C. True – CRH also triggers corticotrope ACTH release.

D. False – It is relatively large, consisting of 41 amino acids.

E. False – They are decreased. It is CSF levels of CRH that are increased.

3.46 Thyrotrophin-releasing hormone (TRH):
   A. Releases prolactin from the anterior pituitary gland.
   B. Is similar in size to CRH.
   C. CSF levels are raised in depression.
   D. Responses (TSH release) are blunted in 50% of patients with major depression.
   E. Is released from the paraventricular nucleus of the hypothalamus.

3.47 In statistics:
   A. The median is greater than the mode in a positively skewed distribution.
   B. The standard deviation of the sample distribution is known as the standard error.
   C. The chi-square test cannot be used for the analysis of qualitative data.
   D. In a normal distribution 95% of the sample lies within two standard deviations of the mean.
   E. The Wilcoxon rank sum test is a non-parametric test.

3.48 In statistics:
   A. In applying the chi-square test if the expected cell frequencies are small then the F ratio can be used instead.
   B. The t-test is used with qualitative data.
   C. The Wilcoxon rank sum test involves ranking data from the largest value to the smallest.
   D. The Mann–Whitney test is a parametric test.
   E. Spearman's rank correlation coefficient is denoted by r.

3.46

   A.   True – Pituitary prolactin is released in response to TRH, vasoactive intestinal peptide and arginine-vasopressin.

   B.   False – TRH is one of the smallest neuropeptides, consisting of three amino acids.

   C.   True.

   D.   True – 20–70% of patients with major depression have a blunted TSH response.

   E.   True – TRH is localized in this and the dorsomedial nucleus of the hypothalamus.

3.47

   A.   True.

   B.   True – It is calculated by dividing the standard deviation by the square root of the sample size.

   C.   False – It is a non-parametric test.

   D.   True – The two parameters of a normal distribution are the standard deviation and the mean.

   E.   True.

3.48

   A.   False – It is the Fisher exact test that is used. The F ratio is calculated in analysis of variance.

   B.   False – It is used with quantitative data.

   C.   False – It is the reverse. Smallest to largest.

   D.   False – It is a non-parametric test. Essentially equivalent to the Wilcoxon rank sum test.

   E.   False – It is denoted by rho (ρ).

3.49 Single Photon Emission Tomography (SPECT):
A. Has better resolution than positron emission tomography (PET).
B. Resolution is affected by signal attenuation and the Compton effect.
C. The isotopes used include Xenon-133 and Technetium-99m.
D. Most of the isotopes used have a half-life of less than 1 minute.
E. Uses iodine-123 labelled ligands to study receptor density.

3.50 Structural neuroimaging findings:
A. There is progressive ventricular enlargement in schizophrenics.
B. There is a reduction in the size of the superior temporal gyrus in schizophrenia.
C. Frontal cortical volume is reduced in affective disorders.
D. Deep white matter hyperintensities are found in elderly depressives.
E. Alcoholism is associated with cerebral and cerebellar cortical atrophy.

3.49

A. False – The reverse is true. Resolution of about 7–8 mm.
B. True.
C. True.
D. False – Half-lives are in excess of 5 hours.
E. True.

3.50

A. False – The enlargement is non-progressive in contrast to Alzheimer's disease.
B. True – Also medial temporal lobe and frontal lobe.
C. True.
D. True – Associated with poor treatment response.
E. True.

Paper 4

4.1 Partial reinforcement:
A. Is more effective than continuous reinforcement.
B. The response rate decreases at the expected time of reinforcement with a fixed interval schedule.
C. Variable ratio reinforcement is the least effective schedule.
D. With a variable interval schedule the response rate does not vary between reinforcements.
E. With a fixed ratio schedule, reinforcement follows a fixed number of responses.

4.2 Perceptual consistency (object constancy) is maintained in changing circumstances with respect to the following:
A. Size.
B. Shape.
C. Lightness.
D. Colour.
E. Location.

4.3 Memory:
A. Long-term declarative memory includes the knowledge of meanings of words.
B. Registration requires attention.
C. Long-term declarative memory includes the memories that concern skills.
D. Memory is functionally highly localized.
E. Long-term declarative memory includes autobiographical memories.

4.1

A. True – And is more resistant to extinction.
B. False – It increases at expected time of reinforcement.
C. False – It is an effective schedule. Fixed interval schedule is poor at maintaining the conditioned response.
D. True.
E. True.

4.2

A. True – Irrespective of distance.
B. True – Irrespective of perspective.
C. True – Irrespective of illumination.
D. True – Irrespective of lighting.
E. True – Irrespective of motion.

4.3

A. True – Declarative–semantic memory.
B. True.
C. False – This is long-term procedural memory.
D. False – It is poorly localized. Specific memories may be highly localized.
E. True.

4.4 Emotions:
  A. Love and fear are primary emotions as described by Plutchik.
  B. According to the James–Lange theory, emotion is secondary to physiological responses.
  C. The Cannon–Bard theory of emotion emphasizes the involvement of the thalamus.
  D. Surprise and contempt are secondary emotions as described by Plutchik.
  E. The James–Lange theory is supported by the fact that emotional changes are faster than physiological responses.

4.5 The following are types of social power as described by French and Raven:
  A. Reason.
  B. Reward.
  C. Expertise.
  D. Referential.
  E. Co-operation.

4.6 Conformity:
  A. Shown by series of experiments conducted by Zimbardo.
  B. Conformity increases with group number.
  C. Vulnerability to conform is less in those that are intelligent.
  D. Conformity bears no relationship to status of individual or that of others.
  E. Vulnerability to conform is greater in those that are expressive.

4.7 In Milgram's experiments on obedience:
  A. Subject's obedience was increased by presence of the experimenter.
  B. Despite being obedient the subject didn't accept the experimenter's sense of right and wrong.
  C. Obedient subjects were unable to challenge the experimenter's morality because of ensuing social awkwardness.
  D. Subject's obedience was increased by perceived authority of experimenter.
  E. College students were assigned roles of prison guards and prisoners.

4.4

A. False – Primary emotions, eight in number: disgust, anger, anticipation, joy, acceptance, fear, surprise, sadness.
B. True.
C. True.
D. False – Secondary emotions: contempt, love, submission, disappointment.
E. False – This is a criticism of the theory.

4.5

A. False.
B. True – Influence is derived from being able to reward.
C. True – Influence is gained by demonstrating knowledge/skills.
D. True – Influence stems from personal charisma, being liked and admired.
E. False.

Note: Others include: authority and coercion.

4.6

A. False – Experiments conducted by Solomon Asch.
B. True – Optimum is group of three.
C. True.
D. False – Perceived high status of others in a group enhances conformity.
E. False – It is less in those that are expressive, socially able and self-reliant.

4.7

A. True – Also by increasing distance from tortured individual.
B. False – Obedience stems for acceptance of experimenter's sense of right and wrong.
C. True.
D. True.
E. False – Such experiments were conducted by Zimbardo.

4.8 With autocratic leadership:
A. Intra-group interactions are aggressive.
B. Interaction with the leader is task-related.
C. In absence of the leader group members abandon the task.
D. Task completion is good.
E. Creative tasks are most likely to be accomplished.

4.9 Raven's progressive matrices:
A. Rely on information recall.
B. Are particularly sensitive to cultural differences.
C. Cannot be used in those with communication difficulties.
D. Involve diagram completion.
E. Use different tests for different age groups.

4.10 Studies regarding intelligence have shown:
A. Intelligence is inversely related to family size.
B. Intelligence is inherited.
C. Intelligence varies with birth order.
D. Intelligence is associated with education.
E. Boys are more intelligent than girls.

4.11 The following are projective tests:
A. Minnesota Multiphasic Personality Inventory (MMPI)
B. Thematic Apperception Test.
C. Rorschach test.
D. Draw-a-person test.
E. Sentence Completion Test.

4.8

A. True.
B. False – It is submissive and attention-seeking.
C. True.
D. True.
E. False – Urgent tasks are best suited to autocratic style of leadership.

4.9

A. False – hence easy to use.
B. False.
C. False – are particularly suited to use in those with communication difficulties.
D. True.
E. True.

4.10

A. True.
B. True – The closer the biological relationship the closer the IQs approximate.
C. True – Inversely.
D. True.
E. False – Boys have a greater range of intelligence than girls.

4.11

A. False – This is an objective test. Test uses specific questions/items and produces a numerical score that can be easily norm-referenced and statistically analysed.
B. True.
C. True.
D. True.
E. True.

Note: Projective tests are based upon the presentation of an ambiguous stimulus to which the individual responds in keeping with their personality. There are no right or wrong answers and the test situation involves the projection of their own needs.

4.12 Piaget's pre-operational stage of cognitive development:
A. Begins at age 5 years.
B. Is divided into pre-conceptual and intuitive stages.
C. Involves comprehension of conservation (reversibility).
D. Involves symbolic play and animism.
E. Leads into the stage of hypotheticodeductive thought.

4.13 A 9-month-old infant:
A. Is able to speak five words.
B. Is not afraid of the dark.
C. Is able to sit unsupported.
D. Manifests separation anxiety.
E. Has begun purposeful behaviour.

4.14 The sick role:
A. Was defined by Parkes.
B. Provides the patient with rights and places them under certain obligations.
C. Exempts the patient from blame.
D. Requires that the patient co-operates in their treatment and management.
E. Is conferred by the doctor.

4.15 In the aetiology of schizophrenia:
A. Bateson highlighted the importance of abnormal communication.
B. Lidz described the schizophrenogenic mother.
C. Fromm–Reichman discovered the importance of expressed emotion.
D. Life events seem not to be significant in terms of onset of illness.
E. The lifetime risk is more than trebled if both parents are affected rather than just one.

4.12
A. False – Spans ages 2–7 years.
B. True – pre-conceptual (2–4 years of age), intuitive (4–7 years of age).
C. False – This takes place in the next stage of development (concrete operational stage).
D. True – Pre-operational stage involves precausal logic, egocentrism, animism and symbolic play.
E. False – Hypotheticodeductive thought is developed in the formal operational stage (age 11 onwards) which follows the stage of concrete operations.

4.13
A. False – Imitates mother's speech and engages in repetitive babbling.
B. False – between 6 and 12 months of age an infant usually develops a fear of height and darkness.
C. True.
D. True – critical period begins age 6 months.
E. True.

4.14
A. False – Parsons described the doctor–patient relationship and within this the social role of doctors and the sick role of patients.
B. True.
C. True – Also excuses them from their normal duties, e.g. work.
D. True – The patient should also desire recovery and take the necessary steps to seek help.
E. True – Diagnoses and defines the illness and legitimizes it.

4.15
A. False – Bateson described the double-bind. Conflicting messages from parents.
B. False – Lidz described marital schism/skew.
C. False – Fromm–Reichman described the schizophrenogenic mother.
D. True – Life events are more significant in relation to relapse and the course of the illness.
E. True.

4.16 The following are neurotic defences:
A. Intellectualization.
B. Introjection.
C. Sublimation.
D. Reaction formation.
E. Denial.

4.17 Hypnosis is associated with:
A. Charcot.
B. Sheldon.
C. Hull.
D. Mesmer.
E. Braid.

4.18 Primary process thinking:
A. Takes place outside of consciousness.
B. Is systematized.
C. Has low tolerance for inconsistency.
D. Is governed by the pleasure principle.
E. Regards and respects logical connections.

4.19 Descriptions of thought disorder proposed by Cameron include:
A. Malapropism.
B. Paraphasia.
C. Loosening of associations.
D. Overinclusion.
E. Metonym.

4.16
A. True – Akin to rationalization this involves the excessive use of intellectual processes to avoid the expression of feelings.
B. False – This is the opposite of projection. It is a form of identification. It is an immature defence.
C. False – Is a mature defence which involves the diversion of socially unacceptable instincts and drives into socially appropriate, creative activities.
D. True – Attitude/behaviour are directed so that they completely oppose underlying unacceptable impulses.
E. False – This is a narcissistic defence involving the unconscious refusal to accept or acknowledge external reality.

4.17
A. True – Influenced Freud.
B. False – Noted for description of body types.
C. True.
D. True – Animal magnetism. Hence mesmerized.
E. True – More specifically neurohypnotism.

4.18
A. True – Takes place unconsciously.
B. False – Lacks organization.
C. False – High tolerance for inconsistency.
D. True – Reality principle governs secondary process thinking.
E. False – This applies to secondary process thinking.

4.19
A. False – Ludicrous misuse of words.
B. False – Substitution of a word or phrase with one that is wrong or distorted.
C. False – Formal thought disorder; described by Bleuler.
D. True – Describes an inability to circumscribe a problem or retain meaningful boundaries.
E. True – An imprecise expression that only approximates to the intended word or phrase.

Note: Others include interpenetration and asyndesis.

4.20 Cranial nerves:
   A. The motor component of the gag reflex involves the vagus nerve.
   B. The facial nerve conducts taste from the posterior one-third of the tongue.
   C. In conduction deafness the Rinne test is positive.
   D. The spinal nucleus of the trigeminal nerve is primarily concerned with proprioception.
   E. The spinal root of the accessory nerve supplies the temporalis muscles.

4.21 Cerebrospinal fluid (CSF):
   A. Is secreted by the arachnoid granulations.
   B. Is almost protein-free.
   C. Flows between the pia mater and arachnoid layers of the meninges.
   D. Is turbid in tuberculous meningitis.
   E. Is clear in neurosyphilis.

4.22 Periaqueductal grey matter:
   A. Is found in the midbrain.
   B. Haemorrhage is associated with thiamine deficiency.
   C. Surrounds the aqueduct of Sylvius.
   D. Stimulation causes pain.
   E. Contains opiate receptors.

4.20

A. True.

B. False – Anterior two-thirds. Posterior one-third is innervated for taste by glosspharyngeal (IX).

C. False – Rinne test positive is normal (conduction in air > bone). In conduction deafness conduction in bone > air = Rinne test negative.

D. False – Spinal nucleus is primarily involved with pain and temperature sensations. Proprioception involves mesencephalic nucleus.

E. False – Supplies trapezius and sternocleidomastoid.

4.21

A. False – CSF is secreted by choroid plexi within the ventricles, and 300–600 ml are secreted per day. It is actively transported back into the blood circulation via the superior sagittal sinus arachnoid granulations.

B. True – It is a clear, colourless blood-filtrate containing relatively small amounts of protein (30–40 mg/100 ml). It also contains glucose (60–100 mg of glucose per 100 ml) and a very small number of white cells, mainly lymphocytes.

C. True – CSF pushes the arachnoid layer against the dura creating the subarachnoid space between the pia mater and the arachnoid.

D. True – The CSF is turbid in bacterial, viral, fungal and tuberculous meningitis.

E. True – The CSF is clear in health, neurosyphilis and Guillain–Barré syndrome. It is bloody in subarachnoid haemorrhage.

4.22

A. True – The periaqueductal grey matter surrounds the third ventricle and the aqueduct of Sylvius in the midbrain.

B. True – Usually caused by alcohol abuse.

C. True.

D. False – Stimulation of the periaqueductal grey matter results in analgesia through the release of endogenous opioids.

E. True.

4.23 The neurochemistry of Alzheimer's disease:
  A. The concentration of somatostatin is reduced.
  B. Hippocampal glutamate is reduced.
  C. There is a reduction in the concentration of choline acetyl-transferase (ChAT).
  D. The concentration of acetylcholinesterase is increased.
  E. Interneurone gamma-aminobutyric acid (GABA) levels are reduced.

4.24 In multi-infarct dementia:
  A. Ventricular enlargement is rare.
  B. Dementia ensues once the volume of brain tissue affected exceeds 100 ml.
  C. Leukoaraiosis is pathognomic.
  D. Hippocampal and thalamic infarction are protective.
  E. The individual is less likely to be emotionally labile than in Alzheimer's disease.

4.25 Early and late-onset familial Alzheimer's disease are associated with the following genes:
  A. Amyloid precursor protein gene on chromosome 21.
  B. Apolipoprotein E gene on chromosome 19.
  C. Presenilin-1 gene on chromosome 14.
  D. Presenilin-2 gene on chromosome 1.
  E. Tyrosine hydroxylase gene on chromosome 11.

4.26 The long-term sequelae of chronic alcohol abuse include:
  A. Optic atrophy.
  B. Pseudobulbar palsy.
  C. Gait disturbance.
  D. Proximal myopathy.
  E. Sensori-motor neuropathy.

4.23

A. True – Somatostatin co-localizes with GABA.
B. True – Cortical glutamate levels are also reduced.
C. True – There is a loss of basal forebrain cholinergic cortical and hippocampal innervation.
D. False – This too is reduced.
E. True.

4.24

A. False – Ventricular enlargement is common.
B. True – And there is usually no detectable cognitive impairment until 50 ml of brain tissue are affected.
C. False – Leukoaraiosis (white matter rarefaction) is found in up to 40% of the normal elderly population.
D. False – Infarction of these areas may in itself lead to dementia.
E. False – Emotional lability is more likely to occur in those with vascular dementia.

4.25

A. True – This codes for a membrane-bound protein. Associated with up to 10% of early-onset Alzheimer's disease.
B. True – This is associated with both early- and late-onset Alzheimer's disease and is probably a susceptibility factor.
C. True – Membrane-bound protein. Found in almost three-quarters of cases of early-onset familial Alzheimer's disease.
D. True – Membrane-bound protein.
E. False – Tyrosine hydroxylase is the rate-limiting enzyme in monoamine synthesis and is possibly associated with affective disorders in particular bipolar disorder.

4.26

A. True.
B. True – Demyelination results in central pontine myelinolysis and this presents with pseudobulbar palsy.
C. True – Cerebellar degeneration particularly affects the vermis and produces gait disturbance.
D. True.
E. True – Alcohol abuse is also associated with other forms of neuropathy (varcular, viral, traumatic).

4.27 The cerebellar cortex contains the following cells:
  A. Golgi cells.
  B. Bipolar cells.
  C. Granule cells.
  D. Horizontal cells.
  E. Basket cells.

4.28 Ptosis is caused by:
  A. Abducens nerve palsy.
  B. Myasthenia gravis.
  C. Pancoast tumour.
  D. Oculomotor nerve palsy.
  E. Optic nerve damage.

4.29 Clinical features of Huntington's disease include:
  A. Irritability.
  B. Tremor.
  C. Dystonia.
  D. Insidious global dementia.
  E. Abnormal saccades.

4.30 Receptors:
  A. Proprioceptors sense position.
  B. Exteroceptors sense the distant environment.
  C. Free nerve endings are sensitive only to vibration.
  D. Nociceptors sense pain.
  E. Phasic receptors are slow to adapt.

4.27
  A. True – Local circuit neurones. Others include basket cells, stellate cells and granule cells.
  B. False – Found in retina.
  C. True.
  D. False – Found in retina.
  E. True.
Note: Purkinje cells are the principal neurones in the cerebellum.

4.28
  A. False – Commonest ocular palsy. Eye deviates towards nose.
  B. True.
  C. True.
  D. True – Eye is also deviated 'down and out'.
  E. False.

4.29
  A. True – Emotional symptoms are common and include depression, anxiety and irritability.
  B. True – Other motor symptoms include dysarthria and an abnormal lurching and contorted gait.
  C. True.
  D. True – Language function and memory are relatively spared.
  E. True.

4.30
  A. True.
  B. False – Exteroceptors such as those in the skin sense the immediate environment whereas telereceptors such as the ears and eyes sense the distant environment.
  C. False – Free nerve endings are sensitive to pressure, touch, pain and temperature.
  D. True.
  E. False – Phasic receptors adapt rapidly. Tonic receptors adapt slowly.

4.31 Generator potential:
- A. Duration is the same as that of action potentials.
- B. Lacks a refractory period.
- C. Undergoes summation.
- D. Exhibits a graded response.
- E. Conduction is passive.

4.32 α_2 Adrenoceptors:
- A. Are G-protein coupled.
- B. Bind Isoprenaline.
- C. Are pre-synaptic autoreceptors.
- D. Mediate pituitary growth hormone release in response to clonidine.
- E. Mediate changes in locus coeruleus activity.

4.33 $5HT_{1A}$:
- A. Mediates buspirone agonist activity.
- B. Mediates ACTH release.
- C. Mediates pindolol antagonism.
- D. Is also known as the $5HT_{2C}$ receptor.
- E. Is coupled to the phosphatidylinositol second messenger system.

4.31

    A. True – Lasts 1–2 ms.

    B. True – Action potential refractory period is 1 ms.

    C. True.

    D. True – Unlike action potentials in which the response is all-or-none.

    E. True – And the amplitude decreases with conduction.

Note: In mechanoreceptors such as the Pacinian corpuscle receptor activation leads to an initial depolarization called the generator potential.

4.32

    A. True – All adrenoceptors are metabotropic (G-protein coupled).

    B. True – Isoprenaline binding differentiates α and β adrenoceptors. Isoprenaline has greater agonist potency at β adrenoceptors than adrenaline or noradrenaline. The reverse is true of α adrenoceptors. Nevertheless, all are adrenoceptor agonists.

    C. True – α_2 adrenoceptors are inhibitory and are found both pre- and post-synaptically.

    D. True – Clonidine is an agonist at these receptors. Growth hormone release is often blunted in depression.

    E. True – α_2 adrenoceptor agonists suppress electrophysiological activity of locus coeruleus noradrenergic neurones.

4.33

    A. True – $5HT_{1A}$ has both pre- and post-synaptic activity. Agonists include buspirone and ipsapirone. Pindolol is an antagonist. It is found in high density in the hippocampus and raphe nuclei.

    B. True – It also mediates hyperphagia and hypothermia.

    C. True – Other antagonists are cyanopindolol and spiroxatrine.

    D. False – It was the $5HT_{2C}$ receptor that was previously called the $5HT_{1C}$ receptor.

    E. False – Like $5HT_{1B}$, $5HT_{1D}$ and $5HT_4$, it is coupled via a G-protein to adenylate cyclase.

4.34 N-methyl-D-aspartate receptors:
A. Are coupled to adenylate cyclase.
B. Have a specific manganese ion binding site.
C. Are permeable to Na^+, K^+ and Ca^{2+}.
D. Possess a phencyclidine binding site.
E. Give rise to fast EPSPs.

4.35 Lithium:
A. Plasma levels are decreased by the carbonic anhydrase inhibitor acetazolamide.
B. Causes dysgeusia.
C. Induced tremor can be treated with propranolol.
D. Toxicity in the elderly usually presents with dysphagia and constipation.
E. Is prescribed in liquid form as a citrate.

4.36 The following statements concerning benzodiazepines are true:
A. Status epilepticus should be treated initially with intramuscular diazepam or diazepam suppositories.
B. Alprazolam is a short-acting benzodiazepine ($T_{1/2}$ less than 25 h).
C. Co-administration of disulfiram decreases the plasma levels of diazepam.
D. Benzodiazepines increase EEG β-activity.
E. Zolpidem is a 3-hydroxy-benzodiazepine.

4.34

A. False – They are ionotropic receptor channels.
B. False – They have a magnesium ion binding site. Binding is voltage dependent and blocks the receptor channel.
C. True – AMPA and Kainate receptors are only permeable to Na^+ and K^+.
D. True – This site also binds ketamine.
E. False – The EPSPs are slow involving calcium-dependent processes.

4.35

A. True – Increases lithium excretion.
B. True – Dysgeusia (impairment of the sense of taste). Lithium has a metallic taste.
C. True – Lithium results in an accentuated physiological tremor which is best treated by titrating the dose of lithium. However, if this is not possible then propranolol or other β-blockers can be prescribed.
D. False – Lithium toxicity usually presents with lethargy, diarrhoea, abdominal pain, nausea and vomiting accompanied by marked tremor, ataxia and visual disturbances.
E. True – Lithium carbonate is prescribed as tablets and lithium citrate is prescribed as liquid/solution.

4.36

A. False – Absorption from either of these is too slow. Diazepam should be administered intravenously, preferably as an emulsion to minimize the risk of venous thrombophlebitis, or as a rectal solution. Alternatively lorazepam or clonazepam can be used.
B. True – Short-acting: alprazolam (12); lorazepam (15); midazolam (2–3); oxazepam (8–10); and temazepam (10). Half-lives in parentheses in hours.
C. False – Disulfiram increases the plasma levels of 2-keto-benzodiazepines (clorazepate, chlordiazepoxide, diazepam and flurazepam).
D. True – Also increase EEG θ activity.
E. False – Zolpidem is an imidazopyridine and not a benzodiazepine, however, it acts on the same group of receptors.

4.37 Phenobarbitone:
- A. Acts as an anticonvulsant by inhibiting GABA-mediated processes.
- B. Is metabolized to primidone an active metabolite.
- C. Elimination is enhanced by the ingestion of activated charcoal.
- D. When used for a long period of time produces a hypochromic microcytic anaemia.
- E. Inhibits a breast-feeding infant's sucking reflex.

4.38 In the treatment of substance abuse:
- A. Diethylthiocarbamate, a metabolite of disulfiram, inhibits dopamine β-hydroxylase.
- B. Lofexidine is used for the symptomatic management of opioid withdrawal.
- C. Rivastigmine is used in opioid dependence to maintain abstinence.
- D. Naltrexone is used in once opioid-dependent individuals to prevent relapse.
- E. Acamprosate is used in the management of alcohol withdrawal.

4.37

A. False – Phenobarbitone acts by enhancing GABA-mediated inhibitory processes.

B. False – Primidone is metabolized to phenobarbitone as is methylphenobarbitone.

C. True – Activated charcoal is used following an overdose or poisoning to both limit the absorption of certain drugs from the gastrointestinal tract and enhance the elimination of others (phenobarbitone, carbamazepine, aspirin).

D. False – Chronic use usually leads to a megaloblastic anaemia because of folate deficiency.

E. True – Breast-feeding is not advised.

4.38

A. True – Disulfiram itself is an aldehyde dehydrogenase inhibitor and the ingestion of alcohol results in the accumulation of acetaldehyde producing an array of unpleasant side-effects.

B. True – Like clonidine it acts centrally to reduce sympathetic tone.

C. False – Rivastigmine is an acetylcholinesterase inhibitor that is used in the symptomatic treatment of mild to moderate dementia in Alzheimer's disease.

D. True – It is an opioid antagonist that is prescribed to former addicts to prevent relapse.

E. False – Acamprosate is used in the maintenance of abstinence in alcohol dependence. It should be prescribed once abstinence has been achieved although treatment can continue even if the patient relapses.

4.39 Psychosurgical procedures used for the treatment of psychiatric disorders:
A. Are associated with an increase in the incidence of seizures.
B. Include subcaudate tractotomy.
C. Are used to treat intractable obsessive–compulsive disorder.
D. Are no longer available in Europe.
E. All necessitate craniotomy.

4.40 Recognized cutaneous features of neurofibromatosis include:
A. Butterfly rash.
B. Axillary freckling.
C. Café au lait patches.
D. Naevus flammeus.
E. Melanoma.

4.39

   A. True – For most procedures there is a modest increase in the risk of seizures. Following stereotactic subcaudate tractotomy the risk at 1 year follow-up is 1–2%.

   B. True – Other currently available procedures include cingulotomy, capsulotomy and limbic leucotomy.

   C. True – Other indications are treatment-resistant depression and intractable anxiety disorders.

   D. False – There are several centres in Europe currently providing psychosurgery.

   E. False – Gamma capsulotomy does not require craniotomy. The gamma knife creates specific lesions by focusing more than 200 beams of cobalt-60 gamma radiation using a helmet-like stereotactic unit.

4.40

   A. False – Found in systemic lupus erythematosus and tuberous sclerosis.

   B. True.

   C. True – They are found in 10% of the normal population. More than five (each greater than 1.5 cm diameter) is abnormal.

   D. False – Port-wine naevus. Found characteristically in Sturge–Weber syndrome.

   E. True.

Note: Other recognized features of neurofibromatosis include renal artery stenosis, aortic coarctation, neural tumours, berry aneurysm, obstructive cardiomyopathy, diabetes insipidus, mesenteric ischaemia, phaeochromacytoma, hypospadias, scoliosis, pulmonary fibrosis, fibrous dysplasia of bone, and local limb gigantism.

4.41 Recognized features of phenylketonuria include:
A. Eczema.
B. Seizures.
C. Polydactyly.
D. Macular cherry red spot.
E. Mousy odour.

4.42 Lesch–Nyhan syndrome:
A. Is an autosomal recessive disorder.
B. Arises because of Hexosaminidase-A deficiency.
C. Is noted for self-mutilating behaviour.
D. Is associated with an increase in head size.
E. Results in the accumulation of mucopolysaccharides in tissues.

4.43 Fragile X syndrome:
A. Occurs in 1 in 1000 of the general male population.
B. Is less common in women than men.
C. Rarely causes mental retardation.
D. Is an X-linked dominant disorder.
E. Is associated with autistic disorder.

4.41

A. True – Also tissues are pigment deficient (blue eyes, blonde hair and fair skin).
B. True – Infant is normal for first few weeks of life. There is then increasing intellectual impairment, cerebral palsy and autistic behaviour.
C. False.
D. False – Macular cherry red spot is found in Tay–Sachs disease.
E. True.

4.42

A. False – It is an X-linked recessive disorder.
B. False – This is the defect in Tay–Sachs disease.
C. True.
D. False – head size is actually smaller than usual.
E. False – It arises because of a deficiency of hypoxanthine phosphoribosyl transferase in purine metabolism.

Note: Its features include choreoathetosis, hyperuricaemia, seizures, spasticity, self-mutilation and small head size.

4.43

A. True – It is the second most common cause of mental retardation in males.
B. True – Occurs in 1:2000 women. Women are usually carriers but can express phenotypical features and have mental retardation.
C. False – Commonly causes mental retardation. The degree of mental retardation is variable.
D. False – It is X-linked recessive. Fragile site [Xq27].
E. True – Also with attention-deficit disorder.

4.44 Prolactin release from the anterior pituitary:
A. Is inhibited by serotonin.
B. Is blunted in response to d-fenfluramine in depression.
C. Is inhibited by phenothiazines.
D. Is diminished by sleep.
E. Is inhibited by arginine-vasopressin.

4.45 Growth hormone release:
A. Is inhibited by pyrexia.
B. Is blunted in response to clonidine in major depression.
C. Peaks with the onset of slow-wave sleep.
D. Is inhibited by somatostatin.
E. Is diminished by opioids.

4.46 The following hypothalamic neurotransmitters inhibit feeding:
A. Neuropeptide Y (NPY).
B. Serotonin.
C. Cholecystokinin (CCK).
D. Noradrenaline.
E. Corticotrophin-releasing hormone.

4.44

A. False – Serotonin and tryptophan indirectly enhance the release of prolactin.
B. True – In depression prolactin release in response to d-fenfluramine, clomipramine and tryptophan is blunted.
C. False – These drugs are D2 antagonists and consequently remove the dopamine-mediated inhibition of prolactin release. This leads to hyperprolactinaemia and side-effects of gynaecomastia, galactorrhoea, amenorrhoea, impotence and infertility.
D. False – Sleep, pregnancy and exercise all increase the release of prolactin.
E. False – Like TRH and vasoactive intestinal peptide (VIP), arginine-vasopressin stimulates the release of prolactin.

4.45

A. False – Growth hormone release is stimulated by pyrexia, hypoglycaemia, exercise, sleep, surgery and stress.
B. True – Clonidine is an α_2 agonist. The responses to desipramine and hypoglycaemia are also blunted in major depression.
C. True.
D. True – It is sometimes referred to as the growth hormone-release-inhibiting-factor.
E. False – Opioids stimulate the release of growth hormone and diminish the inhibitory effect of somatostatin.

4.46

A. False – NPY is one the most potent known appetite stimulants. Opioids also stimulate feeding.
B. True – And serotonin uptake inhibitors are used to reduce weight. Neurotensin also inhibits feeding.
C. True – CCK is linked with satiety.
D. False – Noradrenaline stimulates feeding (α_2 adrenoceptor-mediated effect).
E. True.

4.47 In statistics:
A. For rare conditions the odds ratio approximates to the relative risk.
B. The attributable risk is the incidence of a disease in an exposed group minus its incidence in an unexposed group.
C. The *p*-value is the probability of making a type II error.
D. Non-parametric tests require that variables are measured on a ratio scale.
E. The sensitivity is the proportion of those without the disorder that have a negative test result.

4.48 Functional neuroimaging findings:
A. Hypofrontality in schizophrenia.
B. State-dependent changes in cingulate cortex blood flow in depression.
C. Increased blood flow to parahippocampus in anxiety disorders.
D. Reversible hypofrontality in depression.
E. No functional changes in obsessive–compulsive disorder.

4.47

A. True.

B. True.

C. False – The probability of making a type II error is that of incorrectly rejecting the alternative hypothesis. The *p*-value is the probability of obtaining a significant outcome through chance alone.

D. False – Non-parametric tests can be applied to ordinal and nominal scale measures.

E. False – This is the specificity.

4.48

A. True – N.B. Liddle's symptom clusters.

B. True – Normalize with clinical recovery.

C. False – Reduced blood flow to right parahippocampus and reduced benzodiazepine receptor density in several brain regions.

D. True.

E. False – Functional changes have been found in the caudate nucleus and orbitofrontal cortex. These normalize with clinical recovery.

4.49 *Amanita muscaria* (**fly agaric mushroom**) **contains:**
A. Nicotine.
B. Muscarine.
C. Ibotenic acid.
D. Muscimol.
E. Caffeine.

4.50 Ventricular enlargement in schizophrenia is associated with:
A. Cognitive decline.
B. Decreased frontal cerebral blood flow.
C. Decreased cerebrospinal fluid homovanillic acid.
D. Positive psychotic symptoms.
E. Fewer negative symptoms.

4.49
    A. False.
    B. True.
    C. True.
    D. True – GABA agonist.
    E. False.

4.50
    A. True.
    B. True.
    C. True.
    D. False – Less.
    E. False – More.

Paper 5

5.1 The following statements are true:
- A. Chaining is a learning technique occasionally used in people with learning difficulties.
- B. Flooding is also known as explosion therapy.
- C. Prempack's principle states that naturally occurring high frequency behaviours cannot be further reinforced.
- D. Shaping is based upon operant conditioning.
- E. Sensitization involves gradual exposure to an hierarchy of anxiety-inducing stimuli from least to most.

5.2 The following cues are important in the creation of a three-dimensional percept from a two-dimensional retinal image:
- A. Relative brightness of objects.
- B. Object interposition.
- C. Motion parallax.
- D. Binocular convergence.
- E. Object texture gradient.

5.3 Short-term memory:
- A. Is also described as working memory.
- B. Coding is primarily visual.
- C. Finite capacity of 7 + 2 units of information.
- D. Recall is error-free and effortless.
- E. Capacity can be enhanced by chaining.

5.4 Groupthink:
- A. Leads to the adequate exploration of alternatives.
- B. Is more likely to occur when there is open-ended discussion with few constraints.
- C. Is less likely in the presence of a prominent opinionated leader.
- D. Results in deindividuation.
- E. Is facilitated by shielding the group from outside influences.

5.1

A. True – The desired complex behaviour is broken down into a series of simpler steps which are taught individually and then linked together.

B. False – Flooding is the immediate and sustained exposure to a highly anxiety-inducing stimulus *in vivo*.

C. False – Prempack's principle states that high frequency behaviour can be used to reinforce a low frequency behaviour by making engagement in the former contingent upon satisfying some aspect of the latter.

D. True.

E. False – This describes systematic desensitization. Sensitization involves the strengthening of a response to a stimulus because of its significance.

5.2

A. True.

B. True.

C. True.

D. True.

E. True.

Note: Others include monocular accommodation, relative size, elevation and binocular vision.

5.3

A. True – Also described as primary memory.

B. False – Primarily acoustic.

C. True.

D. True.

E. False – Capacity can be enhanced by chunking.

5.4

A. False – It results in inadequate exploration of alternatives.

B. False – It is more likely to occur when there is pressure to conclude.

C. True.

D. True – This is the suppression of individuality.

E. True.

Note: Groupthink is the tending of group decisions towards consensus with individuals suppressing opposing opinions so as to avoid dissension.

5.5 Aggression:
A. In terms of social learning theory is considered to be a basic instinct.
B. Ethologically, can be diminished through familiarity with the aggressor.
C. Is described as instrumental when its aim is primarily to injure.
D. And aggressive behaviour are diminished by emotional arousal.
E. Is closely associated with frustration.

5.6 The following are associated with aggressive behaviour:
A. Young parents.
B. Permissive parenting.
C. Small family size.
D. Positive emotional expression.
E. Viewing television violence.

5.7 The following statements are true:
A. In minority ingroups the outgroup is perceived as being homogeneous.
B. In majority ingroups the ingroup is perceived as being heterogeneous.
C. In relation to others the members of an ingroup are perceived more favourably.
D. Prejudice stems from differences in attitudes and beliefs.
E. Prejudice and stereotypes are difficult to change.

5.8 Studies have shown that the IQ of children is related to:
A. Social class.
B. Education.
C. Perseverance.
D. Parental wishes.
E. Home life-style.

5.5

A. False – In terms of social learning theory aggression is learnt through modelling. It is ethological theories and psychoanalytical theories that consider aggression to be innate or a basic instinct.
B. True – Also by distancing self and by evoking a conciliatory response.
C. False – Instrumental aggression is aimed at gaining some kind of reward. Hostile aggression is aimed at injury/harm.
D. False – Emotional arousal increases aggressive behaviour.
E. True – Frustration–aggression hypothesis. Failure to achieve causes frustration.

5.6

A. True.
B. True – And inconsistent parenting styles.
C. False – Large families.
D. False – Lack of emotional expression is associated with aggressive behaviour.
E. True – Only in boys.

5.7

A. False – This is true if ingroup is the majority. Converse is true, i.e. outgroup is perceived as heterogeneous.
B. True.
C. True.
D. True.
E. True.

Note: Ingroup: that with which an individual identifies. Outgroup: individual has an association with this group but does not identify with this group.

5.8

A. False.
B. True.
C. True.
D. False.
E. True.

Note: Intelligence has an inverse relationship with increasing family size and birth order. Boys have a greater range of intelligence than girls.

5.9 In Erikson's theory of psychosocial development:
A. A crisis of integrity versus despair occurs in adolescence.
B. There is less emphasis on psychosexual development than in Freud's theories.
C. Epigenesis refers to the stages of ego and social development.
D. The successful resolution of the intimacy versus isolation crisis in adulthood results in commitment.
E. There are no issues of importance in the stage of latency (age 5–12 years).

5.10 Personality:
A. Kretschmer described pyknic body-build as relating to a solitary, self-conscious and aloof personality.
B. Sheldon described those that preferred to enjoy themselves and relax as being of endomorphic body type.
C. Kretschmer's athletic body-build is equivalent to Sheldon's mesomorphic body type.
D. Eysenck described personalities as introverted or extroverted.
E. Cattel's trait theory of personality describes 16 first-order personality factors and three dimensions.

5.11 Piaget's concrete operational stage of cognitive development:
A. Commences at the age CNS myelination is completed.
B. Involves deductive reasoning.
C. Involves adherence to authoritarian morality.
D. Is the shortest stage of development.
E. Involves the development of logic.

5.12 Language is slower to develop in:
A. Girls.
B. Twins.
C. Small families.
D. Deaf children.
E. Immigrants.

5.9

   A. False – This occurs in maturity and successful resolution results in fulfilment.

   B. True.

   C. True.

   D. True.

   E. False – Crises of initiative versus guilt and competence versus inferiority are dealt with. There is no stage of latency.

5.10

   A. False – This describes the asthenic or leptosomatic body type. The pyknic body type is relaxed, sociable, variable in mood.

   B. True – Also called viscerotonic.

   C. True – Outgoing, robust, show energy and assertiveness.

   D. True.

   E. True – Dimensions of anxiety, intelligence and sociability.

5.11

   A. True – Age 7 years.

   B. False – This is achieved in the next stage, that of formal operations.

   C. False – This is a feature of the previous stage (pre-operational).

   D. False – The first stage of development (sensorimotor) is the shortest. The concrete operational stage spans approximately 4 years, ages 7–11.

   E. True – Also develop identity and individuation of thought and comprehend the laws of conservation.

5.12

   A. False – Boys develop language skills later than girls.

   B. True.

   C. False – Development is slower in large families.

   D. True.

   E. False – No evidence for this, however, language is slower to develop in those from social classes IV and V.

5.13 A 3-year-old child:
  A. Understands size (small, big).
  B. Has entered Kohlberg's second level (stages 3 and 4) of moral development.
  C. Is fearful of strangers.
  D. Can distinguish left and right.
  E. Is able to copy a triangle.

5.14 Life events:
  A. Can be assessed objectively using the Holmes and Rahe Social Readjustment Scale.
  B. Are significant in terms of onset of schizophrenia.
  C. Often precede puerperal psychosis.
  D. Are associated with Post Traumatic Stress Disorder (PTSD).
  E. Often precede suicide attempts.

5.15 Goffmann used the following terms to describe the process of mortification:
  A. Colonization.
  B. Betrayal funnel.
  C. Binary management.
  D. Batch living.
  E. Role-stripping.

5.16 The following are immature defences:
  A. Isolation.
  B. Somatization.
  C. Regression.
  D. Splitting.
  E. Identification.

5.13

    A. True.

    B. False – This does not begin until the age of 7 years.

    C. True.

    D. False – This is not usually achieved until aged 4 or 5 years.

    E. False – This is not usually achieved until the age of 6 years.

5.14

    A. False – This is a self-report questionnaire. A more reliable and valid measure is the semi-structured interview (Life Events and Difficulties Schedule–LEDS).

    B. False – Only in terms of relapse and course of illness.

    C. False – No such relationship has been found in studies.

    D. True – By definition PTSD involves a significant life-event.

    E. True.

5.15

    A. False – Part of the reaction to mortification, involves pretence of compliance.

    B. True – Describes the role of relatives that send the patient to hospital with the help of health professionals.

    C. False – Refers to the differences between the environments of staff and patients.

    D. False – Refers to the absence of the normal components of life.

    E. True – for example, removal of personal effects.

5.16

    A. False – This is a neurotic defence involving the separation of an idea from its original associated affect (which has been repressed).

    B. True – Psychological phenomena are expressed as bodily symptoms.

    C. True – At times of stress the individual unconsciously retreats to an earlier level of emotional functioning.

    D. False – This is a narcissistic defence and involves an inability to integrate opposing aspects of personality.

    E. True – The unconscious adoption of desirable attributes of others.

5.17 Sigmund Freud:
  A. In his topographical model of the mind described the conscious, preconscious and subconscious.
  B. Supplanted the topographical model with the structural model of the mind in which he described the id, ego and superego.
  C. Developed the concentration method.
  D. Published 'studies on hysteria'.
  E. Analysed Sandor Ferenczi.

5.18 The following are associated with hysteria:
  A. Cade.
  B. Briquet.
  C. Charcot.
  D. Janet.
  E. Hecker.

5.19 The following types of hallucinations are correctly described:
  A. Functional: those caused solely by non-organic illnesses.
  B. Autoscopic: visual hallucination of oneself.
  C. Reduplicative: black and white visual hallucinations (lack colour).
  D. Hypnopompic: occur at time of going to sleep.
  E. Experiential: visual hallucinations occurring in temporal lobe epilepsy.

5.20 The following statements are correct:
  A. Athetosis is absent during sleep.
  B. Automatic obedience is also called command automatism.
  C. Mitmachen is a form of automatic obedience.
  D. Mitgehen is an extreme form of mitmachen.
  E. Ambitendency is a disorder of gait.

5.17

   A. False – He used the term unconscious not subconscious defining it as all mental processes outside of consciousness.

   B. True.

   C. True – This followed his use of the technique of hypnosis.

   D. True – In 1895 in conjunction with Breuer.

   E. True – Ferenczi described active therapy and forced fantasies.

5.18

   A. False – Noted for use of lithium.

   B. True.

   C. True – Influenced Freud.

   D. True – Also psychasthenia.

   E. False – Noted for description of hebephrenia.

5.19

   A. False – Both the normal percept and the hallucination that it produces are simultaneously perceived.

   B. True.

   C. False – Experience of an additional limb or body part.

   D. False – At time of waking up. Hypnogogic when going to sleep.

   E. True.

5.20

   A. True.

   B. True – Individual behaves in any manner that is requested regardless of any consequences.

   C. True – Individual despite being requested to resist allows their body to be freely positioned.

   D. True.

   E. False – Individual is unable to complete an action, repeatedly starting and stopping.

5.21 Nystagmus is associated with:
  A. Wernicke–Korsakoff syndrome.
  B. Phenytoin.
  C. Labyrinthitis.
  D. Vertebrobasilar artery occlusion.
  E. Multiple sclerosis.

5.22 The following result in atrophy, paresis and diminished reflexes:
  A. Spinal cord damage.
  B. Diabetic peripheral neuropathy.
  C. Poliomyelitis.
  D. Stroke.
  E. Pseudobulbar palsy.

5.23 The following occur in REM sleep:
  A. Night terrors.
  B. Bruxism.
  C. Sleep-walking.
  D. Sleep myoclonus.
  E. Nightmares.

5.24 The pathology of Alzheimer's disease includes:
  A. Hippocampal pyramidal cell granulovacuolar degeneration.
  B. Loss of pyramidal neurones from cortical layers III and V.
  C. Astrocyte proliferation.
  D. Cortical Lewy bodies.
  E. Hirano bodies.

5.21

A. True.

B. True – Can occur at therapeutic doses.

C. True.

D. True.

E. True.

5.22

A. False – Upper motor neurone damage results in clonus, spasticity, hyperactive deep tendon reflexes.

B. True – This affects lower motor neurones.

C. True.

D. False.

E. False.

Note: Atrophy, paresis and diminished reflexes are signs of lower motor neurone damage.

5.23

A. False – Night terrors usually occur in children and occur during slow-wave sleep (Stages II and IV).

B. False – Grinding of the teeth (bruxism) occurs during non-REM sleep.

C. False – Occurs in non-REM sleep.

D. False – Periodic movements in sleep. Associated with restless legs syndrome. Occurs during non-REM sleep.

E. True.

5.24

A. True – The appearance of dense granule containing vacuoles.

B. True.

C. True.

D. False – These are found in Parkinson's disease and Lewy body dementia.

E. True – Hirano bodies are rod-shaped eosinophilic cytoskeletal abnormalities that also occur in normal ageing.

5.25 The pathology of idiopathic Parkinson's disease includes:
A. Increased cortical noradrenaline.
B. Locus coeruleus depigmentation.
C. Increased substantia nigra substance P.
D. Reduced frontal cortex somatostatin.
E. Reduced cerebellar cholecystokinin.

5.26 Recognized features of Lewy body dementia include:
A. Parkinsonism.
B. Neurofibrillary tangles.
C. Senile plaques.
D. Loss of neurones from substantia nigra.
E. Fluctuating cognitive state.

5.27 In the retina:
A. The ganglion cell layer consists of cell bodies.
B. There are two plexiform layers.
C. The axons of bipolar cells form the optic nerve.
D. The fovea is free of photoreceptors.
E. Rod- and cone-mediated perception is called mesopic vision.

5.28 Horner's syndrome is associated with:
A. Anhidrosis.
B. Lateral medullary (Wallenberg's) syndrome.
C. Mydriasis.
D. Lack of pupillary light reflex.
E. Cervical spinal cord injury.

5.29 In patients with AIDS cerebral lesions are produced by the following:
A. Toxoplasmosis.
B. Kaposi's sarcoma.
C. Lymphoma.
D. Tuberculosis.
E. Cryptococcus.

5.25

A. False – Cortical noradrenaline and that in the locus coeruleus is reduced.
B. True – Cells in the substantia nigra, vagus dorsal motor nucleus and locus coeruleus undergo depigmentation.
C. False – This is reduced.
D. True.
E. False – It is substantia nigra cholecystokinin that is reduced.

5.26

A. True – Characteristic triad of parkinsonism, fluctuating cognition and recurrent visual hallucinations.
B. True.
C. True.
D. True – Also observe neuronal loss from basal nucleus of Meynert and locus coeruleus.
E. True.

5.27

A. True – The other layers that are principally cell bodies are the inner and outer nuclear layers.
B. True – Inner and outer, both of which contain the synapses and processes of cells.
C. False – It is the axons of the ganglion cells that form the optic nerve.
D. False – It is free of rods but still has cones.
E. True – Photopic and scotopic vision refer to that mediated by cones and rods, respectively.

5.28

A. True.
B. True.
C. False.
D. False.
E. True.

5.29

A. True.
B. True.
C. True.
D. True.
E. True.

5.30 Features of *both* Down's syndrome and Alzheimer's disease include:
- A. Dementia.
- B. Neurofibrillary tangles.
- C. Chromosome 21 associated abnormality.
- D. Amyloid plaques.
- E. Reduction in cerebral acetylcholine.

5.31 Characteristic eye signs of Wilson's disease include:
- A. Macular cherry red spot.
- B. Aniridia.
- C. Sunflower cataract.
- D. Brushfield's spots.
- E. Retinal phakomas.

5.32 Generator potential amplitude:
- A. Diminishes with conduction of the potential.
- B. Determines action potential amplitude.
- C. Varies according to the intensity of the stimulus.
- D. Is sensitive to adaptation.
- E. Is sensitive to stimulus rate of change.

5.33 Vanadium:
- A. Is an essential trace element.
- B. Inhibits sodium–potassium ATPase.
- C. Is an effective antidepressant.
- D. Blood levels are reduced in depression.
- E. Concentration is increased with ascorbic acid.

5.34 *N*-methyl-D-aspartate receptors:
- A. Bind polyamines.
- B. Bind zinc ions.
- C. Possess glycine binding sites.
- D. Interact with AMPA receptors.
- E. Are unaffected by alcohol.

5.30
- A. True.
- B. True.
- C. True.
- D. True.
- E. True.

5.31
- A. False – This is found in Tay–Sachs disease.
- B. False – This is associated with Wilm's tumour.
- C. True – Affects the lens because of copper deposition. Copper deposition in the cornea on the outer margin of the iris produces Kayser–Fleischer rings.
- D. False – Associated with Down's syndrome.
- E. False – Found in tuberous sclerosis.

5.32
- A. True – This is because conduction is passive.
- B. False – It only determines action potential frequency.
- C. True.
- D. True.
- E. True.

Note: Sensory transduction is amplitude-dependent. Transmission of information is frequency-coded.

5.33
- A. True.
- B. True.
- C. False.
- D. False.
- E. False.

5.34
- A. True – Spermidine and spermine. Polyamines can either facilitate or inhibit NMDA receptor function.
- B. True – Binding results in voltage-independent blockade.
- C. False – These sites are insensitive to strychnine and allosterically modulate NMDA receptor function.
- D. True – AMPA receptor-mediated depolarization results in the activation of NMDA receptors.
- E. False – At concentrations producing intoxication alcohol inhibits excitatory amino acid receptor function.

5.35 The GABA$_A$ receptor:
A. Is a ligand-gated chloride ion channel.
B. When competitively blocked raises the seizure threshold.
C. Binds benzodiazepines.
D. Mediates fast post-synaptic EPSPs.
E. Consists of seven membrane spanning proteins.

5.36 The glycine receptor:
A. Is a ligand-gated chloride ion channel.
B. Is excitatory.
C. Binds strychnine.
D. Is modulated by glutamate AMPA receptors.
E. $\alpha 1$ subunit is mutated in human familial startle disease (Kok's disease).

5.37 Carbamazepine:
A. Is an effective mood stabilizer.
B. Is structurally related to tricyclic antidepressants.
C. Acts as an anticonvulsant by inhibiting GABA aminotransferase.
D. Is useful in the treatment of trigeminal neuralgia.
E. Elimination is enhanced by activated charcoal.

5.35

A. True – It is an ionotropic receptor permeable to Cl ions.
B. False – Blockade produces convulsions.
C. True – Also barbiturates, anaesthetic steroids and ethanol.
D. False – IPSPs not EPSPs.
E. False – It consists of five glycoprotein subunits that form the chloride channel.

5.36

A. True.
B. False – Glycine is an inhibitory amino-acid transmitter synthesized primarily from serine. The receptor is responsible for glycine-mediated hyperpolarization.
C. True – Derived from the Strynos seed, strychnine is a potent glycine receptor antagonist that can cause muscle stiffness, convulsions and death.
D. False – Glutamate NMDA receptors possess a glycine binding site and it is these receptors that interact with AMPA receptors.
E. True – Also called hyperekplexia the disease is an inherited mutation of the $\alpha 1$ subunit. The individual falls when startled because of muscular rigidity.

5.37

A. True – It is often used in the treatment of bipolar disorder.
B. True – It is an iminostilbene.
C. False – It acts by limiting the repetitive firing of sodium-dependent action potentials. Vigabatrin inhibits GABA aminotransferase.
D. True – During the acute stages of the illness. Phenytoin is also of use.
E. True.

5.38 Procyclidine:
A. Is useful in the treatment of tardive dyskinesia.
B. Can be administered orally, intramuscularly and intravenously.
C. Is useful in the treatment of drug-induced dystonia.
D. Is effective in treating bradykinesia.
E. Causes sialorrhoea.

5.39 Zuclopenthixol:
A. Is not available as an antipsychotic depot injection.
B. Can be administered intramuscularly, as an acetate, for the short-term management of acute psychosis.
C. Is a piperidine side-chain phenothiazine.
D. Is formulated for oral use as zuclopenthixol dihydrochloride.
E. Is indicated for use in the treatment of depressive illness.

5.40 The following antidepressants block noradrenaline re-uptake:
A. Trazodone.
B. Reboxetine.
C. Venlafaxine.
D. Mirtazapine.
E. Nefazodone.

5.38

A. False – Antimuscarinic agents aggravate tardive dyskinesia and attempts have been made to treat tardive dyskinesia with cholinergic agents such as arecholine and acetylcholine precursors (lecithin, choline, deanol) with limited success.

B. True – As can benztropine.

C. True.

D. False – The antiparkinsonian effects of antimuscarinic agents are only moderate, with respect to tremor and rigidity, and minimal with respect to bradykinesia.

E. False – the opposite is true. Causes dryness of the mouth.

5.39

A. False – Zuclopenthixol can be administered orally, in tablet form (dihydrochloride) or intramuscularly as an acetate or decanoate.

B. True – More commonly referred to as 'acuphase'.

C. False – It is a thioxanthene-like flupenthixol.

D. True.

E. False – It is flupenthixol that has recognized antidepressant effects and is prescribed in low doses for this purpose.

5.40

A. False – Trazodone is a $5HT_2$ antagonist and serotonin re-uptake inhibitor. It is also an antagonist at histamine and α_1 adrenergic receptors.

B. True – Reboxetine is a selective noradrenaline re-uptake inhibitor.

C. True – Sometimes called a dual re-uptake inhibitor, venlafaxine inhibits the re-uptake of both serotonin and noradrenaline.

D. False – Mirtazapine is not a re-uptake inhibitor, instead it blocks pre-synaptic α_2 adrenoceptors and in doing so enhances serotonergic and noradrenergic transmission.

E. True – Its main effect is that of $5HT_2$ antagonism, however, it is also a serotonin and noradrenaline re-uptake inhibitor and an antagonist at α_1 adrenoceptors.

5.41 The blood–brain barrier:
  A. Is absent in neonates.
  B. Includes capillary endothelium.
  C. Is readily permeable to oxygen and carbon dioxide.
  D. Is absent in the area postrema.
  E. Is readily permeable to dopamine.

5.42 Features of tuberous sclerosis include:
  A. Epilepsy.
  B. Ash-leaf spots.
  C. Adenoma sebaceum.
  D. Mental retardation.
  E. Shagreen patches.

5.43 Recognized features of Fragile X syndrome include:
  A. Small low set ears.
  B. High-pitched perseverative speech.
  C. Disproportionately tall stature.
  D. Prognathism.
  E. Macro-orchidism.

5.41

A. False.
B. True – It consists of astrocyte end feet, the basement membrane and capillary endothelium.
C. True – Glucose also readily crosses the blood brain barrier (BBB) although it uses a specific transport mechanism to do so. Most psychotropic medications are lipid soluble and cross the BBB.
D. True – It is also absent because of capillary vessel fenestration in hypothalamic regions, the pineal body, choroid plexi and hypophysis.
E. False – Hence the use of L-dopa (dopamine precursor) in the treatment of Parkinson's disease.

5.42

A. True – Usually intractable.
B. True – Hypo-pigmented areas (amelanotic naevi) that are best viewed with Wood's light.
C. True – Firm, uniformly pale nodules of several millimetres in diameter that occur on the malar surface of the face.
D. True – Cognitive decline may begin in childhood and progress slowly.
E. True – Leathery, flesh-coloured, scaly, lumbo-sacral plaque-like lesions.

5.43

A. False – The ears are characteristically large and 'floppy'. They are often low-set.
B. True – Often described as nasal.
C. False – They are of noticeably short stature.
D. True.
E. True.

5.44 Rett's disorder:
- A. Is diagnosed clinically in the first few weeks of life.
- B. Manifests only in females.
- C. Is associated with macrocephaly.
- D. Rarely results in seizures.
- E. Leads to the development of stereotyped behaviours.

5.45 In major depression:
- A. More than 90% of patients exhibit dexamethasone non-suppression.
- B. Hypercortisolaemia rarely normalizes with clinical recovery.
- C. Adrenal gland volume is increased.
- D. Pituitary gland volume is diminished.
- E. ACTH and cortisol responses to ipsapirone are blunted.

5.46 Plasma levels of the following are significantly reduced in anorexia nervosa:
- A. Oestrogen.
- B. Cortisol.
- C. Cholecystokinin (CCK).
- D. Free thyroxine (T_4).
- E. Growth hormone.

5.44

A. False – Development is normal for the first 6 months of life and diagnosis is made clinically as the child begins to display characteristic features of the disorder.

B. True – It is an X-linked dominant disorder that in males is presumably incompatible with life.

C. False – Growth of the head progressively slows, resulting in acquired microcephaly.

D. False – These are a salient and common feature, occurring in 75% of cases.

E. True – Hand-washing, wringing and clapping.

5.45

A. False – Dexamethasone non-suppression is found in 50–70% of major depressives and 90% of those with psychotic depression. It is non-specific and is also found in dementia, OCD, eating disorders, and up to 10% of the normal population.

B. False – Hypercortisolaemia occurs in about 50% of patient with major depression and usually normalizes with clinical recovery.

C. True – Shows 70% increase with MRI.

D. False – There is usually pituitary gland enlargement.

E. True.

5.46

A. True – gonadotrophin levels are also lowered.

B. False – There is hypercortisolaemia.

C. False – CCK levels are increased.

D. False – The levels of free T_4 are normal however total T_4 and tri-iodothyronine (T_3) levels are low.

E. False – Growth hormone levels are increased.

5.47 Glucocorticoid receptors:
   A. Are also called type I steroid receptors.
   B. Have greater affinity for cortisol than mineralocorticoid receptors.
   C. Are more widely distributed than mineralocorticoid receptors.
   D. Are involved in hypothalamic–pituitary–adrenal axis negative feedback.
   E. Are not found outside the central nervous system.

5.48 In statistics:
   A. The Poisson distribution is a continuous probability distribution.
   B. The coefficient of kurtosis is a measure of dispersion.
   C. A negative coefficient of skewness applies to a distribution with a tail to the right.
   D. The normal distribution is also called the Gaussian distribution.
   E. Yates' Correction applies to the Chi-squared distribution.

5.49 The following are correctly paired:
   A. Imprinting and Konrad Lorenz.
   B. Experimental neurosis and Ivan Pavlov.
   C. Bereavement and Jean Piaget.
   D. Epigeneis and John Bowlby.
   E. Surrogate mother and Harry Harlow.

5.50 The vertebral arteries and their branches supply the following:
   A. Vermis.
   B. Internal capsule.
   C. Occipital lobe.
   D. Frontal lobe.
   E. Broca's area.

5.47

A. False – They are referred to as type II receptors.
B. False – They have less affinity for cortisol than type I receptors.
C. True – Mineralocorticoid receptors are found mainly in the septo-hippocampal complex.
D. True.
E. False.

5.48

A. False – Like the binomial distribution it is a discrete distribution.
B. False – It assesses shape, specifically 'peakedness' of a distribution.
C. False – The reverse is true.
D. True.
E. True.

5.49

A. True.
B. True.
C. False.
D. False.
E. True.

5.50

A. True.
B. False.
C. True.
D. False.
E. False.

Suggested reading

Standard textbooks

It is important to select a suitable standard text that covers most the subject matter in one volume. These books will have to be read repeatedly and essentially learnt, particularly for their clinical content. You only need *one* book and this should be one with which you are comfortable, that is, find easy to read and understand.

- Kendell, R.E. and Zealley, A.K. (eds) (1998) *Companion to Psychiatric Studies*, 6th edn. Edinburgh: Churchill Livingstone.
- Murray, R., Hill, P. and McGuffin, P. (1997) *The Essentials of Postgraduate Psychiatry*, 3rd edn. Cambridge: Cambridge University Press.
- Gelder, M., Gath, D., Mayou, R. and Cowen, P. (1996) *Oxford Textbook of Psychiatry*, 3rd edn. Oxford: Oxford University Press.

Psychopathology texts

Choose *one* only. Although the oldest one of these books is arguably the best, the most recent is most easily available and possibly the most relevant to current examinations and practice.

- Sims, A. (1995) *Symptoms in the Mind*, 2nd edn. London: W.B. Saunders.
- Kräupl-Taylor, F. (1979) *Psychopathology: its Causes and Symptoms*, revised edition. Sunbury-on-Thames: Quartermaine House.
- Hamilton, M. (1974) *Fish's Clinical Psychopathology. Signs and Symptoms in Psychiatry*, revised reprint. Bristol: Wright.

Basic science texts

Each of these books has different strengths. Examine all of them but be selective. Choose *one*.

- Trimble, M. (1996) *Biological Psychiatry*. Chichester: Wiley. (Most up-to-date).
- Morgan, G. and Butler, S. (1993) *Seminars in Basic Neurosciences*. London: Gaskell. (Easiest to use).
- Weller, P. and Eysenck, M. (1992) *Scientific Basis of Psychiatry*. London: W.B. Saunders. (Classic text).

Additional texts

These can be used for reference purposes but will be needed relatively frequently.

- Bland, M. (1995) *An Introduction to Medical Statistics*. Oxford: Oxford Medical Publications.
- Silverstone, T. and Turner, P. (1995) *Drug Treatment in Psychiatry*, 5th edn. London: Routledge.
- *British National Formulary*, latest edition. (An essential text).
- Atkinson, R.L., Atkinson, R.C., Smith, E. and Bern, D. (1993) *Introduction to Psychology*, 11th edn. San Diego: Harcourt Brace.
- Brown, D. and Peddar, J. (1991) *Introduction to Psychotherapy*, 2nd edn. London: Routledge.
- Malhi, G. S. and Bridges, P. K. (1998). *Management of Depression*. London: Martin Dunitz.
- Malhi, G. S., Matharu, M. S. and Hale, A. S. (2000). *Neurology for Psychiatrists*. London: Martin Dunitz

Reference texts

These are useful texts but probably not worth investing in for the purposes of the examination and should be used for clarification and further reading.

- Lishman, W.A. (1998) *Organic Psychiatry*, 3rd edn. Oxford: Blackwell Science.
- Brown, R. (1994) *An Introduction to Neuroendocrinology*. Cambridge: Cambridge University Press.

- McKenna, P.J. (1994) *Schizophrenia and Related Syndromes.* Oxford: Oxford University Press.
- Paykel, E.S. (1992) *Handbook of Affective Disorders*, 2nd edn. Edinburgh: Churchill Livingstone.
- Checkley, S. (1997) *The Management of Depression.* Oxford: Blackwell Science.
- Walsh, K. (1994) *Neuropsychology, a Clinical Approach.* Edinburgh: Churchill Livingstone.

Subject Index

Note: Question numbers are given instead of page numbers